Psychoanalysis and the Wisdom of Ecclesiastes

"Paul Marcus brings Ecclesiastes and psychoanalysis together in mutually fruitful ways. He brings out a "double structure" in Ecclesiastes characterized by profound ambivalence and ambiguity that creatively interacts with psychoanalysis in co-nourishing ways. Whether it is the psychology of wisdom, hedonism, work or love, Marcus opens significant experiential possibilities that add to our sense of being, inviting deep study and amplification."

– **Michael Eigen, Ph.D.,** Author, *Contact with the Depths, Faith, and Kabbalah and Psychoanalysis*

"This original study takes the reader through the book of Ecclesiastes, revealing its conceptual framework and probing its reflections on human existence. Throughout, Marcus brings to bear his unique psychoanalytical perspective, enabling him to suggest new approaches to understanding this important biblical book."

– **Lawrence H. Schiffman,** Global Distinguished Professor of Hebrew and Judaic Studies, New York University

Psychoanalysis and the Wisdom of Ecclesiastes looks at one of the most profound books in the Hebrew Bible – Ecclesiastes, known as Koheleth in Hebrew – through a psychoanalytic lens.

Paul Marcus explores Ecclesiastes' understanding of the profound and compelling problematics of the human condition and explains how he offers a sensible and feasible attitude toward contemporary life. Comparing Ecclesiastes' way of looking at life to the Freudian worldview, Marcus suggests what psychoanalysis might in part appropriate or further explore and develop as it tries to enhance itself as a narrative of the human condition and a compelling "technology of the self." The book also uses psychoanalysis to illuminate aspects of Ecclesiastes that have been underappreciated and undercomprehended.

Psychoanalysis and the Wisdom of Ecclesiastes will be of interest to psychoanalysts exploring spirituality and the human condition, and to academics and students of psychoanalytic studies, religious studies, Judaic studies, and philosophy.

Paul Marcus is a training and supervisory analyst at the National Psychological Association for Psychoanalysis in New York City and co-chairperson of the discussion group Psychoanalysis and Spirituality at the American Psychoanalytic Association. He is the author/editor of 25 books including *The Spiritual Resistance of Rabbi Leo Baeck: Psychoanalysis and Religion* (Routledge). He is currently the editor of *Psychoanalytic Review*.

Routledge Focus on Mental Health

Routledge Focus on Mental Health presents short books on current topics, linking in with cutting-edge research and practice.

Being a Crisis Chaplain
Delivering Help and Healing in Critical Scenarios
Sidney Dekker and Lance Mergard

A Critical Examination of Irvin D. Yalom's Single Session Consultations
It Is the Relationship That Heals
Windy Dryden

The Power of Being a Subject
Transcending Human Mechanics with Critical Thinking, Honesty, Patience, and Bravery
Matthew H. Bowker

The Knowledge of the Psychoanalyst
Raul Moncayo

Elements of Faith: Psychoanalytic Phenomenon and Lived Experience
Brent Potter

The Power of Being a Subject: Transcending Myth and Machine
Matthew H. Bowker

Psychoanalysis and the Wisdom of Ecclesiastes: A Time to Heal
Paul Marcus

For more information about this series, please visit: www.routledge.com/Routledge-Focus-on-Mental-Health/book-series/RFMH

Psychoanalysis and the Wisdom of Ecclesiastes

A Time to Heal

Paul Marcus

Routledge
Taylor & Francis Group
LONDON AND NEW YORK

First published 2026
by Routledge
4 Park Square, Milton Park, Abingdon, Oxon OX14 4RN

and by Routledge
605 Third Avenue, New York, NY 10158

Routledge is an imprint of the Taylor & Francis Group, an informa business

British Library Cataloguing-in-Publication Data
A catalogue record for this book is available from the British Library

ISBN: 9781041099765 (hbk)
ISBN: 9781041099772 (pbk)
ISBN: 9781003652816 (ebk)

DOI: 10.4324/9781003652816

Typeset in Times New Roman
by Apex CoVantage, LLC

For Irene

Recently published Routledge titles by Paul Marcus

The Spiritual Resistance of Rabbi Leo Baeck (2025)
Psychoanalysis and Wisdom. Encountering 'Ethics of the Fathers' (2024)
Psychoanalysis and Toileting. Minding One's Business (2023)
Psychoanalysis as a Spiritual Discipline. In Dialogue with Martin Buber and Gabriel Marcel (2021)
Psychoanalysis, Classic Social Psychology and Moral Living. Let the Conversation Begin (2020)
The Psychoanalysis of Overcoming Suffering. Flourishing Despite Pain (2019)
The Psychoanalysis of Career Choice, Job Performance, and Satisfaction. How to Flourish in the Workplace (2017)

Contents

Acknowledgments *viii*

1 Introduction: A Time to Heal 1

2 Koheleth's General Worldview 7

3 Summary of Ecclesiastes 17

4 The Futility of Wisdom 32

5 The Futility of Hedonism 44

6 The Futility of Work 55

7 The Futility of Love 64

8 Implications for Psychoanalysis 77

References *83*
Index *89*

Acknowledgments

I would like to thank Professor Knut Martin Heim for his reading and critiquing of my book. Thanks also go to my wife, Irene, a child and adult psychoanalyst, for her helpful comments on the manuscript. I am also grateful to Michael Eigen and Lawrence H. Schiffman for their promotional endorsements of my book. Thanks also go to editor Susannah Frearson for her support of my writing project and to Saloni Singhania, her editorial assistant. I alone am responsible for the contents of this book.

1 Introduction

A Time to Heal

The great author of Moby Dick, Herman Melville, regarded Ecclesiastes as "the truest of all books" (Ryken, 2015, p. 4), while the American novelist Tom Wolf characterized Ecclesiastes as "the highest flower of poetry, eloquence and truth – the greatest single piece of writing I have known" (Ryken, 2015, p. 133). Indeed, Old Testament scholar Professor Knut Martin Heim called Ecclesiastes "a magnificent prophetic and poetic masterpiece" (2019, p. 10).

This book looks at one of the most profound, subversive, and beautiful books in the Hebrew Bible, Ecclesiastes, known as Koheleth ("member of the assembly," "Preacher," "Teacher") in Hebrew.[1] Koheleth does not present a consistently thought-out system or logical structure in his reflections; rather, in his brief talks, parables, maxims, and proverbs, we are presented with a series of free associations on the meaning of existence,[2] the good that man can achieve in life and the problematics of finding or creating an enduring sense of personal happiness.[3] Specifically, Koheleth contains the melancholy, skeptical, ironic, and rationalist reflections of a philosopher-poet at the sunset of his life rather than a straightforward, unambivalent pious affirmation of faith and the virtues of living a religious life. Not only does Koheleth strongly question some of the core beliefs in Jewish tradition and its worldview, but most important for this book, he raises many of the most profound questions about human experience and conduct for life that have been of concern to most serious thinkers for thousands of years, including in our time, to psychoanalysis.

Most recently, Heim (2019) for example, characterizes Ecclesiastes as an instance of political satire and a clandestine form of humor. He describes the book as being full of self-parody and as "hilarious" in some places (p. 190). Heim's view, however, is a minority one (Heim, personal communication). I will take up Koheleth's "tragicomic" outlook in Chapter 2.

There are many very good translations of Koheleth. I have opted for Gordis (1951), which I found the most accessible. Lohfink (2003) indicated in his excellent commentary that Gordis' commentary "is one of the best commentaries ever written on Koheleth" (p. ix). Likewise, Murphy (1992) described Gordis' translation and commentary as one of the "great ones of the past" (Preface). Perry (1993) says that Gordis' commentary is "still of great value"

DOI: 10.4324/9781003652816-1

(p. 50). Other notable translations include Crenshaw (1987), Perry (1993), Seow (1997), Longman (1998), Fox (1999, 2004), Bartholomew (2009), Alter (2010), and Heim (2019). It is worth mentioning that "scholars do not agree about its provenance, language, literary genre, unity, or overall message" (Kugel, 1996, p. 258). As Murphy noted in his fine commentary, "No other book in the Bible has so steadfastly defied analysis and refused to be typed" (1992, Preface).[4]

My argument in this book is that, as one of the most illustrious of the "Wisdom" writers, those ancient professional teacher-sages who were committed to developing "a realistic approach to the problems of life, including the practical skills and the technical arts of civilization" (Gordis, 1951, pp. 16–17), Ecclesiastes not only identifies, with dazzling brilliance and poetic perceptiveness, some of the most profound and compelling problematics of the human condition as modern humanity conceives it, but also offers what I believe is in many ways a sensible and feasible attitude toward contemporary life ("a sane, workable attitude toward life," (Gordis, 1951, p. 18)).[5] Moreover, Ecclesiastes' way of looking at life is not only similar to certain life attitudes, beliefs, and values embodied implicitly in the Freudian worldview (and other schools of psychoanalytic thought) (Marcus and Rosenberg, 1998), but also possibly suggests what psychoanalysis might in part appropriate or further explore and develop as it tries to enhance itself as a narrative of the human condition and a compelling "technology of the self."

For example, Ecclesiastes emphasizes that we are deeply relational beings, spending most of our time navigating the different stages of our relationships and the impacts they have on us (Gibson, 2017). Relational analysts have claimed similarly.

In other words, Ecclesiastes provides us with some of the most illuminating and insightful reflections on modern existence and our sense of what, for many, ultimately matters in life (what the existentialists call the problem of Meaning, Ecclesiastes is a forerunner of existential philosophy). Psychoanalysis, as it is concerned with self-transformation and creative and reasonable life-conduct, can only benefit from an engagement with this at times angst-ridden, but always courageous, truth seeker and lover of life in Jerusalem. This being said, psychoanalysis can also illuminate aspects of Ecclesiastes that have been underappreciated and comprehended. For example, Koheleth's state of mind and how we can account for it (Root, 1889; Zimmermann, 1973).

Who Was Ecclesiastes?

There is vast and divergent scholarly literature on Ecclesiastes. Both the more skeptical and pious have found support for their preferred interpretation. Briefly, as noted by Robert Gordis – in my view, one of the seminal scholars on Ecclesiastes – the Book of Ecclesiastes was written in Hebrew by a Jew residing in Jerusalem who knew Aramaic but no Greek, though he was knowledgeable about certain Greek ideas such as the "golden mean" (Gordis, 1951, pp. 68, 22, 78). "Hence do not be righteous overmuch nor be overzealous for wisdom – why be left desolate?" (Gordis, 1951, p. 168).[6] The book was written towards the end of Koheleth's life, about 250 BCE, which correlated with the experience of national defeat, humiliation, and subjugation, between about the fifth to the second centuries. Scholars have inferred that Ecclesiastes was probably something of a country gentleman, a bachelor with no children who probably came from what can be described as a comfortable upper-middle-class background with a socially and politically conservative outlook. The tradition of the Synagogue, however, assumes, incorrectly according to most scholars, that it was none other than Solomon, the son of David, who wrote the Book of Ecclesiastes (Zlotowitz, 1994).[7] As Seow (1997) notes, "The most important reason for the acceptance of the book [in the sacred canon] was that the early interpreters found it possible somehow to interpret the document as orthodox" (such as the last six verses that affirm God and doing His commandments) (p. 4).

Koheleth was one of the professional teachers of Hebrew Wisdom, one manifestation of the literary genre that was part of the social world of the Fertile Crescent, which existed in Egypt, Babylonia, Syria, and Palestine during the second and first millenia BCE (Gordis, 1951, p. 9). Ecclesiastes probably taught in one of the well-to-do local academies that educated upper-class Jewish male youth. Wisdom literature is the most secular branch of ancient Hebrew literature, compared to Torah (with its focus on the practical and exacting obligations of living a pious and God-fearing life) and Prophecy (which focused on the ethical perfection of the Jewish nation and social justice). Wisdom literature, as Hebrew Bible scholar R.B.Y. Scott has pointed out, in general "taught a practical philosophy through which the men might find satisfaction in life in a moral order which had established itself through experience" (Scott, 1965, pp. 202–203).

While Hebrew Wisdom had its antecedents in more ancient cultures (e.g., Egypt, Phoenicia, and Mesopotamia) and neighboring groups (e.g., Edomites), there are basically two main kinds of Wisdom literature, which embodied the contrasting attitudes among the Jewish sages (Scott, 1965, pp. xviii, xix). The first is exemplified in the Bible by the Book of Proverbs. It tends to be conservative, pragmatic, didactic, optimistic, and worldly wise. It sought a rational comprehension of human existence and a foundation for ethics, through the use of reason to observable data and experience. The second type is highly critical, almost rebellious, in its attitude toward traditional beliefs. The second type of Wisdom literature tends to be theoretical, individualistic, and pessimistic. Ecclesiastes, like Job, is in the second group (Scott, 1965, p. 96).

While Koheleth believed in God, for it was inconceivable at that time for a Jew to do otherwise (though not exactly the conventional God of his time), his focus as a Wisdom teacher was on the problems of individual existence and experience. That is, on the difficulties of finding and creating an existentially tolerable if not meaningful life and attaining a degree of personal happiness – all within the context of certain deeply troubling "facts" of human existence. For example, the transitory nature of life, the certainty of death, and man's sense of helplessness before an ultimately unfathomable and uncontrollable universe. Koheleth, like Freud, is characterized by his unshakable intellectual honesty, his courageous use of reason in facing the most agonizing problems of life, his absolute refusal to sureness where he saw ambiguity and uncertainty, and the relentless devotion to truth, regardless of the uncomfortable ramification in one's personal life (Gordis, 1951, pp. 37–38). Moreover, like Freud, Koheleth was attempting to reconfigure his subjectivity, to fashion a self and autonomous and self-governing being, both within the context of the parameters of the society in which he lived and in terms of what he took to be the limitations inherent in being (and in Koheleth's case, in terms of the seeming limitations and enigmas in God's relationship to humanity).

Finally, as I will attempt to suggest, like Freud at his best, Koheleth was committed to a relentless critique of himself and his main mode of self-fashioning. Koheleth questioned nearly all of the taken-for-granted social paradigms and interpretations of self that were operative at his time, and in this sense, he was, to some extent, attempting to fashion a new form of life that departed from the coercive normalizing institutions of priestly scribes and orthodox theologians within his community. Lastly, as I will suggest, like Freud, Koheleth ended up, in part, advocating an attitude toward life characterized by resignation without despair, combined with an unwavering commitment to striving after joy in life, fleeting as these joyful experiences may be.

The Book of Ecclesiastes is overflowing with provocative ideas about life, love, suffering, growing old, and death, and it is impossible in this book to discuss all of them. I therefore will focus on a few of the major themes that embody his "philosophy of life," as it were, and seem to be most relevant to psychoanalysis.

What Is Psychoanalysis?

I conceptualize psychoanalysis as a form of life, a meaning-giving, affect-integrating, and action-guiding resource for individuals who can appropriate the life- and identity-defining narrative of psychoanalysis when they seek to understand, endure, and possibly gain some mastery of the problems that affect, if not assault, the human experience of love, work, faith, and suffering (e.g., conflict, anxiety, despair, loss, and tragedy). As philosopher Pierre Hadot notes about ancient Greek philosophy, psychoanalysis can be understood as a "spiritual exercise," a tool for living life skillfully, more fully and wisely (1997, p. 83). The aim of a spiritual exercise is to foster a deep modification of an individual's way of "seeing and being," a decisive change in how one lives one's practical, everyday life. Michel Foucault (a student of Hadot's) also discussed spiritual exercises, calling them "technologies of the self": "an exercise of the self, by which one attempts to develop and transform oneself, and to attain a certain mode of being" (Foucault, 1989, p. 433). Most importantly, the objective of a spiritual exercise is "a total transformation of one's vision, life-style, and behavior" in the service of increased personal freedom and equipoise (Hadot, 1997, pp. 14, 83, 103) and, I would add, a less self-centric outlook and behavior. According to this view, as Levinas described "Jewish humanism" at its best, psychoanalysis is "a difficult wisdom concerned with truths that correlate to virtues" (1989, p. 275).

Psychoanalysis is a painful, deconstructive, demythologizing, and defamiliarizing process for acquiring greater self-awareness and self-understanding, especially of one's destructive unconscious emotional activity, one that transforms moral consciousness by expanding and deepening one's capacity to love. As Freud suggested, at least ideally, self-understanding leads to self-mastery, which leads to self-transcendence of one's impediments to being more other-directed, other-regarding, and other-serving (i.e., less crudely narcissistic and in other ways neurotically self-absorbed). In fact, Freud described psychoanalytic treatment as the "scientific cure by love" (McGuire, 1974, pp. 12–13). In this sense, psychoanalysis is animated by both the "love of wisdom" and the "wisdom of love," by Greek and Hebrew values (Levinas, 1981, p. 162), and is a powerful tool for the art of living a good life as one construes and fashions it.

This book is organized as follows. Chapter 2, on Koheleth's general worldview, attempts to give a snapshot of his perspective on life. The book of Ecclesiastes is characterized by a double structure. Koheleth, for example, is optimistic, then pessimistic, life-denying, and then life-affirming, a man of many contradictions. Ambivalence and ambiguity are his hallmark. Indeed, Koheleth is a highly conflicted elderly man who left many unclarified passages in his narrative. Chapter 3, a summary of Koheleth, provides a synopsis of each of the 19 sections of the book of Ecclesiastes as organized by Gordis (1951). This chapter is meant to familiarize the reader with the content and major themes of the book. Chapter 4, the futility of wisdom, drills down deeper into why Koheleth found wisdom so deficient in his search for deep and abiding meaning. Psychological definitions of wisdom are discussed and their psychoanalytic significance are suggested. Chapter 5, the futility of hedonism, discusses why Koheleth found pleasure-seeking inadequate as a way of life. "Responsible pleasure-seeking" is introduced into Koheleth's outlook and psychoanalytically explored. Chapter 6, the futility of work, focuses on Koheleth's criticisms of those who make work the absolute center of their life. The differences between a job, career, and calling are described and psychoanalytically probed. Chapter 7, the futility of love, drills down deeper into Koheleth's belief that love both does and does not provide a basis for a coherent narrative of self-identity. Love is discussed in terms of the work of Sigmund Freud, Erik. H. Erickson, Melanie Klein, Heinz Kohut, and Jacques Lacan. Chapters 4, 5, 6, and 7 have a clinical case vignette that correlates with the main themes of the chapter. Finally, Chapter 8, implications for psychoanalysis, discusses how psychoanalysis can benefit from an in-depth study of Ecclesiastes as well as what psychoanalysis can offer to enhance the theory and practice of psychoanalysis.

Notes

1 I will refer to the book of Ecclesiastes as Ecclesiastes while I will use the name Koheleth as the author.

2 As Alter (2010) notes, Kohelet's "thought is freewheeling and associative" (p. 342). As Weeks (2020) points out, "Qohelet is not a comedian, but his monologue resembles many modern stand-up routines, moving as they do through different topics with a mixture of anecdotes, one-liners and maybe even poems" (p. 13).

3 Recently, there has been an explosion of empirical research on happiness. In fact the *New York Times* did a whole issue devoted to the science of happiness (*New York Times Magazine*, The Happiness Issue, 5/4/2025). One of the major conclusions was that it takes more than material prosperity to produce true flourishing; in general, social connectivity matters more (Johnson et al., 2025).

4 All translations have their limitations. For example, translation difficulties emanate from linguistic and cultural differences, such as idioms, slang, and the nuances of language structure, in addition to technical knowledge divergencies and temporal constraints. Also, one's interpretive frame impacts translations. As the great literary critic George Steiner wrote somewhere, "Every translation is a world."

5 Recently, the existence of a "genre" of Wisdom Literature has been called into question: See Keynes (2019). It is too early to know how much traction this challenge will gain, but for our purposes, it is unlikely that the essential characteristics of Ecclesiastes explored here will change significantly (Heim, Personal communication).

6 Koheleth is mindful of the dangers of excess, whether good or evil. He observes that extreme virtue potentiates self-righteousness, and excessive vice imperils one's life (Crenshaw, 1987).

7 When Koheleth calls himself the "king over Israel in Jerusalem," he adopts the persona of King Solomon as a "literary device" (Gordis, 1951, p. 138). The book is told by an unnamed narrator who probably wrote the introduction and epilogue, though Fox (1999) believes there may be an implied third voice. Bartholomew (2009) believes that the voices of the narrator and the implied author are one and the same. Also, there may not be a historical Koheleth, his name being a nickname or pseudonym, possibly for the narrator who he speaks through. The book's straightforward religious ending, affirming God and keeping his commandments, is probably one of the reasons that it was made part of the sacred cannon by the ancient Rabbis. Ecclesiastes is read in the synagogue during the Sabbath of Succoth, the feast of Booths, probably because of its invitation to rejoice (Lohfink, 2003).

2 Koheleth's General Worldview

Koheleth is the consummate *homo viator*, what the existentially oriented Christian philosopher Gabriel Marcel called a spiritual wayfarer or traveler. Koheleth has written an intensely personal self-study, a "reflective autobiography" (Fox, 1999, p. 155), one that is suffused with ambivalence and ambiguity.[1] In fact, it is precisely the highly conflictual and contradictory nature of his experiences that characterizes what Gordis calls Koheleth's "world-view" (Gordis, 1951, p. 112). Other prominent Koheleth scholars also refer to Koheleth's conflicted worldview such as Murphy (1992, p. xliii), Fox (2004, p. xxix), Alter (2010, p. 343), and Heim (2019, p. 135).

In this chapter I want to give an overview of this worldview, while the chapters that follow will look at some specific issues in greater detail, such as the futility of wisdom, hedonism, work, and love.

I will structure this overview chapter in terms of regarding Koheleth as something of an analysand in treatment. As I do in analysis, I am highly sensitive to how the analysand problematizes his life, what he regards as troubling, in terms of him asking himself three concrete and practical questions: What is the problem? How did it get there? How to "fix" it? Gordis (1951) also organizes his analysis of Koheleth by asking three questions: What is Kohelelth rejecting and complaining about? What is he affirming and recommending? What are the underlying reasons for each? (p. xxv). Likewise, in accordance with Gordis, Fox (2004) claims that all interpretations of Ecclesiastes must answer the same three fundamental questions: What is Koheleth negating and complaining about? What is he affirming and recommending? What are his underlying reasons for each? (p. xxv).

Before summarizing Koheleth's worldview, I want to define what I mean by worldview and suggest its limitations as a concept, as it applies to Koheleth's largely "free associations." Free association was the basis of Freud's self-analysis and he instructed his analysands to speak without censoring their thoughts (Akhtar, 2009). As I will suggest here, some have argued that psychoanalytically speaking, having a worldview is itself the problem! (Bass, 1998).

DOI: 10.4324/9781003652816-2

A worldview, says psychologist Koltko-Rivera, is defined as follows:

> A way of describing the universe and life within it, both in terms of what is and what ought to be. A given worldview is a set of beliefs that includes limiting statements and assumptions regarding what exists and what does not (either in actuality, or in principle), what objects or experiences are good or bad, and what objectives, behaviors, and relationships are desirable or undesirable.

Moreover,

> a worldview defines what can be known or done in the world, and how it can be known or done. In addition to defining what goals can be sought in life, a worldview defines what goals should be pursued. Worldviews include assumptions that may be unproven, and even improvable, but these assumptions are super ordinate, in that they provide the epistemic and ontological foundations for other beliefs within a belief system.
>
> (2004, p. 4)

As psychoanalyst Alan Bass (1998) has noted, Freud was against the idea of a psychoanalytic Weltanschauung (worldview) in part because it is antipsychoanalytic, that is, it went against the basic thrust of psychoanalysis, which following Freud is that "it cannot be systematic."[2] Philosophers, theologians, and psychotics, according to Freud, strive for systematicity, but psychoanalysis should not, in part, because it fundamentally concerns itself with "unconscious energic processes" that by definition are contradictory, paradoxical, and ambiguous and therefore must challenge our habitual conscious patterns of organizing data. In other words, for Bass, like Freud, to seek out or create a Weltanschauung is to succumb to an "illusory wish fulfillment." A commitment to such systematization is not only a form of imprisonment, but it also misses some of the essential themes of psychoanalysis that suggests what Freud thought constituted aspects of the human condition: for example, that human consciousness is inescapably ambiguous and contradictory. Psychoanalysis, says Bass, must push against the tendency to mold itself into the habitual patterns of conscious experience; against Weltanschauungen, it should strive to be more like an endless movement that perpetually undoes itself (Marcus and Rosenberg, 1998, editor's introduction, pp. 412–413).[3] As Freud said, "Philosophy sometimes seems to me like a person who keeps cleaning their glasses and they still stay dim" (https://www.freud.org.uk › Blog Accessed 2/25/25).

Freud was not entirely consistent in his views on philosophy. He wrote for example, that "our art consists in making possible for people to be moral and to deal with their wishes philosophically" (Hale, 1971, p. 121).

While being mindful of Bass's critique of the notion of worldview, I will attempt to characterize not so much Koheleth's worldview as it is typically understood, but rather in terms of it being the free associations of an ambivalent and ambiguous elderly man as he looks back on his remarkable life. That is, I will attempt to avoid the tendency for "narrative smoothing" in these matters. By narrative smoothing I mean "smoothing out" discrepancies or seemingly immaterial details to generate a more coherent and comprehensible story by eliminating what is regarded as needless information, and organizing the remaining elements in a logical sequence, making it considerably easier to interpret and present the narrative to the reader. Indeed, Koheleth is a highly conflicted elderly man who left many unclarified passages in his narrative. This is one of the reasons the book is so intriguing and charming. "Absolute consistency is not his purpose" (Alter, 2010, p. 340). As Bartholomew (2009) wrote in his excellent commentary on Ecclesiastes, regarding "Ecclesiastes' structure, message, and relationship to the Old Testament traditions and international wisdom, there is no consensus" (p. 40).

It should be stressed from the onset that Koheleth was a religious Jew, that is, being an atheist or agnostic was not typically part of the ancient episteme, the socio-intellectual reality, the thought world that Koheleth was lodged in. However, Koheleth was not a conventional religious believer; in fact he never mentions God's name, YHWH ("The Lord"), throughout his book. He uses the generic designation *Elohim* ("God or gods"). God, says Loader (1986), appears as distant and remote to Koheleth. Koheleth, like Job, had some serious questions about God's relationship to men, such as the fact that an omnipotent, omniscient, omnipresent, and most importantly, all-good God appears to not intervene in the pained lives of those who serve Him (and therefore make things "feel" better). This being said, according to Alter, Kohelet "has enough of a connection with tradition that he never absolutely denies the idea of a personal god" (2010, p. 341). There is a degree of "reverence before the numinous, the *tremendum*," in his way of experiencing the world (Murphy, 1992, p. lxv).[4]

As I have said, Koheleth is, in fact, the quintessential ambivalent, ambiguous man. Somewhat like a neurotic analysand, he is infused with contradictions. Indeed, Crenshaw (1987) and Fox (1999), for example, detail these contradictions. Next are some of the contradictions that Koheleth mentions that characterize his dialectical relationship to truth as he conceives it. Where modernity puts forth the claim that truth exists and that the scientific method is the only reliable way to determine that truth (hence, its rationalist presuppositions), the postmodern view that I am sympathetic with views truth as a subjective construct that is negotiated and varies across cultures and time. Here are 20 illustrative issues that, in part, constitute Koheleth's "high-conflict" worldview. These high-conflict entries will give the reader a good sense of Koheleth the man and his outlook:

1. Koheleth is religious but has his serious misgivings (e.g., God is just, but the world is full of injustices). However, at the end of the book he (or an

editor who wrote the last six verses) attempts "to motivate his contemporaries to remain faithful to their God and their traditional cultural values" (Heim, 2019, p. 8). Says Koheleth, "Fear God and keep His commandments, for that is man's whole duty" (Gordis, 1951, p. 190).[5]

2. Koheleth is a hedonist, yet he is also self-denying.
3. God has inserted in man a drive for happiness; however he can never satiate this drive.
4. Human actions are preordained by God, yet man tries to find/create absolute, ultimate truth (or he lives as if he has acquired such truth). That is, man is helpless "before the mystery of the world," God's inscrutable nature (Gordis, 1951, p. 163).
5. Like a good Marxist, Koheleth says man desires wealth, yet it can never be satisfied in a sustained manner (i.e., most people want more and more).
6. Man tends towards extremes, of saintliness (e.g., fighting for justice) and wickedness (in the Bible roughly equated to folly), yet episodic happiness typically requires living in the "gray zone," the realm of moral half-tints.
7. Death appears to be the terminating point of one's activities (e.g., Koheleth does not dwell on the afterlife or the underworld), yet he quests after immortality. Following psychiatrist Robert Jay Lifton, this can possibly include "symbolic immortality," an "experiential transcendence," that intense feeling where "time and death disappear" (Lifton, 1976, pp. 33–34).
8. Man strives for wisdom, but he is rarely appreciated in his time. In addition, wisdom can be subverted by one act of folly or wickedness. "Don't count a man happy until the day he dies," said the ancient Greek political philosopher Solon.
9. Man does not know when he will be struck down by wickedness, and yet he spends enormous efforts trying to discern and predict such scenarios.
10. Said Koheleth, "Be warned: of making [reading] many books there is no end, and much study wears one's strength away" (Gordis, 1951, p. 191).[6] Speculations, critical self-reflection, may be thought-provoking, but the "life of the mind" can undermine one's motivation to intervene in the "real" world.
11. Koheleth bemoans that the wise man dies as well as the fool, and thus he hates life (2:16–17). On the other hand, he loves life, "a live dog is better than a dead lion" (9:4) (Murphy, 1992).
12. Kohelelth affirms the universality of mortality saliency, of death, yet he is depressed about human mortality (Fox, 2004).
13. Kohelelth asserts that he prefers death to life; however, he also affirms the intrinsic value of living (Fox, 2004).
14. Koheleth, probably a bachelor, articulates a negative if not demeaning view of women whom he did not trust, yet he claims that it is best to be with a woman you love and not be alone (Fox, 2004).

15. Koheleth is prone to entertaining a dialectic, such as between love and melancholy, frustration and resignation, truth and righteousness (Gordis, 1951).
16. Koheleth was a socially conservative intellectual, who dislikes authority, including governmental authority, though he is no revolutionary. He accepts the status quo though he bemoaned the lack of justice in the world (he cannot imagine a just society). However, he never imagined or desired changes in social structure (Fox, 2004), structural variables, or social design.
17. "The words of the wise spoken softly . . . are heeded more that the ruler's shouts are among fools." However, while this is a plausible principle, "To Koheleth's chagrin [it] is often violated" (Fox, 2004, p. 66).
18. Koheleth strives for a permanence in his life in a world that is always changing. Said the ancient Greek philosopher Heraclitus, "You cannot step into the same river twice."
19. Koheleth craves transcendence, yet he appears to be wedded to his everyday routines.
20. Koheleth believes everything is vanity, and yet his epilogist believed that one should fear God and keep his commandments.

As I will suggest throughout this book, Koheleth never really resolves these existential tensions but resigns himself to these challenges, but without deep and abiding despair (or without "too much" despair). Koheleth's technology of the self is similar to Freud's, who regarded the "voice of reason" (probably a Greek influence) to be his main tool in his psychological toolbox for engaging the problem of meaning-maintenance or neurosis (Fox, 2004):

> The boldest, most radical notion in the book is not Koheleth's contradictions, his pessimism,[7] or his observations of injustices. It is the belief that the individual can and should proceed toward truth by means of his own powers of perception and reasoning: and that he can in this way discover truth previously unknown.
>
> (Fox, 2004, p. xi)

From what I can tell, Koheleth does not typically look for Truths with a capital "T." He appears to believe that this is beyond human capacity of perception and cognition. In his "language game" God is fundamentally inscrutable but worth devoting one's life to understanding and serving. The "secret of life" (i.e., the search for Meaning) is not obtainable (Gordis, 1951, p. 112). Rather, what Koheleth ultimately strives for are "usable truths," that is, truths that are context-dependent and setting-specific and that are pragmatically relevant to the particular circumstances that one finds oneself in. As Gordis says, Koheleth is clearly aware that he does not have "a monopoly on the truth" (p. 114). Having a "gods eye" view of Truth, a kind of immaculate perception, appears to be impossible. Koheleth here anticipates a post-modern outlook.

So How Does Koheleth Generally View the World?

As Longman (1998) notes in his splendid commentary, Koheleth was not satisfied simply stating that everything is meaningless or absurd, in addition, he addresses specific domains and suggests why they have no value for him. For example, toil, another name for work, does not bring about lasting satisfaction:

> Someone might work hard and succeed, but then die and have to leave it all to someone who has not worked for it (2:17–23). Furthermore, the motivation to work hard itself is evil because it springs from envy.
>
> (Longman, 1998, p. 32)

Said Koheleth, "I saw that all hard work and skill are merely one man's rivalry with his neighbor" (Gordis, 1951, p. 150, IV. 4–16).

Koheleth provides something of an "antidote" to the aforementioned which I will detail in the chapter on the futility of work. While he emphasizes the importance of work to have a balanced and reasonable life (4:5), he also emphasizes the need to have a peaceful life without work being one of its central pillars (4:6) (Longman, 1998, p. 32). Workaholism was ill-conceived, ill-advised, and ill-fated. For Freud, however, famously noted, "What should a normal person be able to do?" He replied, "He should be able to love and work" (Allport, 1937, p. 275).

Koheleth also affirms the world as meaningless due to the oppression and domination, if not tyranny, that he perceives all around him (4:1–3). He notes that the government is largely responsible for much of the suffering that people have to contend with. One can look at the past diabolical situation of civil war in Syria under Bashar al-Assad, and elsewhere, to know this is often the case. Moreover, as of 2020, there are 52 nations (out of 195) with a dictator or authoritarian regime ruling the country. Koheleth, like so many of us today, feels sympathetic to the resisters, but he is largely resigned to this dismal state of affairs (Longman, 1998). That is, Koheleth is a "teacher and thinker," not "a prophet or guerilla warrior" (Lohfink, 2003, p. 13). His overall comportment is one of "a radical philosopher" (Alter, 2010, p. 3).

Rather surprisingly for a wisdom writer in Israel, Koheleth's attitude toward wisdom (i.e., skill and know-how, good sense) is rather blunted in terms of its significance as compared to folly (i.e., foolish absurdity). That is, while initially in his musings he sounds rather similar to the teachings of Proverbs, claiming that wisdom is superior to folly in that it helps a person effectively navigate everyday life, this advantage of wisdom peters out since whether wise or foolish, in the end, both have the same fate, namely, they die (Longman, 1998). As I will point out in a later chapter, this is only one way of conceptualizing mortality saliency.

Koheleth's quest for meaning leads him to consider the domains of political power, riches, large families, and a long life, finding all of these to be ultimately frustrating and unsatisfying. They are so because of two facts of human existence that are the basis of his ordeal of suffering: that we all die and "the inability to control and know the appropriate time to do anything" (Longman, 1998, p. 33). Says Koheleth, "Everything has its appointed time, and there is a season for every event under the sky" (Gordis, 1951, p. 144, III. 1–15). The problem with this outlook is that one does not know specifically what the right time or right thing to do is – only God knows this, and this is beyond human understanding. As a result of this fact pattern, being at the mercy of time and chance, "life under the sun," everyday living, feels futile (i.e., ephemeral and unreliable (Seow, 1997)). Said Koheleth, "Who knows what is good for man in life, during the brief days of his vain existence, which he spends like a shadow? Who can tell what will happen under the sun after he is gone" (Gordis, 1951, p. 162, VI. 10–12).

Mortality saliency is a key notion for Koheleth, the fact that we humans know we are going to die, and as a result of this fact, all of life feels futile. As Koheleth notes about death, the dead are hardly remembered, certainly without the freshness of detail. "For the living know they will die, but the dead know nothing. There is no longer any reward for them, for the memory of them is forgotten" (9:5, Longman, 1998, p. 226). While there are pleasures of life to enjoy, like eating, drinking, and moderate work, Koheleth believes that there is hardly a difference between humans and animals since they both have the same fate – they die. As Longman notes, Koheleth's main philosophical message is, "Life is full of trouble and then you die" (Longman, 1998, p. 34).[8]

Tragicomic Outlook

Some have claimed that Koheleth has what I would call a tragicomic outlook, seeing the comic in the tragic and the tragic in the comic (Marcus, 2013). For example, Heim (2019) suggests that the book of Ecclesiastes is a form of "political satire," "a clandestine form of humour," a subversive book that can be described as "resistance literature" (pp. 3, 5, 6). He further says, much of Koheleth's "humour is of a dark nature" (Heim, 2019, p. 148). Likewise, Fox (2004) sees a degree of humor in the book, describing Koheleth as "facetiously" speaking (p. 52), as "poking fun at himself" (p. 53), as sounding "ironic" (p. 40), "cynical" (p. 54), "sardonic" (p. 62), and "wry" (p. 71). Gordis (1951) discusses Koheleth's "amused doubts" (p. 113), while Seow (1997) refers to Koheleth's "parody" (p. 50).

While Fox does not make the claim that Koheleth is typically characterized as the aforementioned, there does seem to be a tragicomic "feel" to some of what Koheleth is trying to convey. After all, he does declare that there is "a time to weep and a time to laugh" and "a time to mourn and a time to dance" (Gordis, 1951, p. 144, III. 1–15).

Tragicomedy, says sociologist Peter L. Berger, can be defined "as that which provokes laughter through tears. It is mellow, forgiving. It does not bring about a profound catharsis, but it is moving nonetheless. Above all, it consoles. The consolation may or may not have religious overtones." Moreover, says Berger,

> Tragicomedy differs from benign humor, which, as far as possible, banishes the tragic from the tragic constructions of an artificial reality. . . . So called black humor defies the tragic . . . Then there is grotesque humor, in which the tragic is absorbed into an absurd universe, as the *danse macabre* of the late Middle Ages. In the tragicomedy, the tragic is not banished, not defied, not absorbed. It is, as it were, momentarily suspended.

And finally, Berger notes,

> Tragicomedy like benign humor, often inserts itself in small, fugitive dosages into the flow of everyday life. It does not eradicate whatever sorrow or sadness has obtruded, but it makes these emotions more bearable. Also like benign humor, it is often mediated by children. The vibrant vitality of children is obviously incongruent with whatever may be the tragic situation. The incongruence is comic, but it also reaffirms the power of life in the face of all that darkens the human condition.
>
> (Berger, 1997, pp. 117–118)

Berger uses "Jewish humour" as his main template of the tragicomic at its best. He focuses on the popular Yiddish writer Sholom Aleichem, creator of the lovable but pained character Tevye the Milkman, immortalized in the musical *Fiddler on the Roof.* Aleichem's Tevye (or Koheleth?) is an "unforgettable blend of resignation" without despair, "irony, and the determination to survive against all odds" (Berger, 1997, p. 121). Thus, as with Tevye and Koheleth, it is the capacity of "making light of things, even as his heart is weeping inside him," that beautifully depicts the tragicomic vision that Koheleth subtly and episodically expresses.

Koheleth's Relationship to God

Koheleth did not have traditional Jewish faith, nor did he believe that justice would prevail the way the Prophets claimed. He also did not believe in a hereafter or messianic coming as suggested in Pharisaic Judaism. In addition, and perhaps most importantly, he maintained the impossibility of grasping the meaning and purpose of life. Of course, trying to fathom the meaning of life is like asking a chess master what is the best move in a chess game. He will tell you that it depends on the circumstances one finds oneself. Koheleth appears to not grasp this important postmodern point, that there is no Meaning in life, only meanings depending on the context and setting one is lodged in. This being said, Koheleth, steeped in a traditional background and outlook, never doubted the existence of God for a moment. However, God was unfathomable, and his relationship to men was one of utter perplexity.

While largely rejecting a traditional Jewish outlook, Koheleth was left with a huge problem, how to justify his existence and navigate life's swings and roundabouts.

The one thing that Koheleth seemed to believe in was that the purpose of life was to achieve a modicum of happiness. In his quiet loneliness and haunting sadness (Gordis, 1951), Koheleth engages in a spiritual odyssey that has resonated with his readers for thousands of years. With justice in human affairs an illusion (e.g., good people suffer, bad people prosper), and truth unattainable (e.g., an absolute law of moral cause and effect being elusive; Shields, 2006, p. 15), Ecclesiastes is left with very little upon which to fashion a world of meaning. As I have said, for Koheleth all that is certain is that man has an innate desire for happiness. Since God has created man, He has also created this impulse. It thus becomes clear that God's fundamental purpose for mankind is the furthering of man's happiness. Thus, the basic theme of Ecclesiastes is its insistence upon the enjoyment of life, of all good things in the world. "I know there is no other good in life but to be happy while one lives. Indeed, every man who eats, drinks and enjoys happiness in his work – that is the gift of God" (Gordis, 1951, p. 146, III. 1–15); "Enjoy life with the woman who you love. Through all the vain days of your life. Which God has given you under the sun" (Gordis, 1951, p. 114, 9:9). Exactly what constitutes enjoying life will be unpacked in a future chapter using clinical and other examples.

We may put this point another way: Koheleth's metaphysics postulates the existence of God, combined with His creative power and limitless dominion. But beyond these attributes, Koheleth refuses to affirm anything about his God, except that He has revealed His will to His creatures by embedding in man an ineradicable desire for happiness (notice the divine irony, of inserting in man a drive which he can never satiate). Koheleth's morality accordingly recognizes the pursuit of happiness as the goal. His religion is the combination of his theology and his ethics. One scholar called Ecclesiastes "a theology of happiness" (Heim, 2019, p. 10). It is noteworthy that Freud agreed with Koheleth that happiness was the goal of life: "[What] [do] men themselves show by their behavior to be the purpose and intention of their lives . . . ? The answer to this can hardly be in doubt. They strive after happiness; they want to become happy and to remain so" (Freud, 1930, p. 76).

Notes

1 Seow (1992) describes Ecclesiastes as a "fictional royal autobiography" (p. 48).

2 In this context, says philosopher Emil L. Fackenheim, "a Weltanschauung requires: cosmic scope, internal coherence . . . and a sincere commitment on the part of devotees" (1996, p. 155).

3 Another way of saying this, with a religious sensibility like Koheleth's, is that "a closed system cannot endure transcendence" (Rotenstreich, 1968, p. 162).

4 Longman (1998) claims that for Koheleth, "God's purpose is to frighten people. In Qohelet's estimation, he is a cosmic bully" (p. 132). This is in tension with what the other scholars think, more extreme.

5 Most biblical scholars think that the third person account is an epilogue, in which the editor summarizes Koheleth's teaching with these words (Heim, personal communication).

6 Again, most scholars believe this is the Epilogist speaking.

7 Koheleth's pessimism is evident, for example, in his conviction of the transience of man, uselessness and repetition of things that occur, and human forgetfulness (Loader, 1986).

8 Koheleth is not the first human to discover that we die. It is not clear what makes this knowledge more devastating for him than for most. Longman does not deal with this issue. From my clinical experience, people who find the fact that they are going to die as devastating often have control issues, which leads to obsessing over the finality of life. They can't give up "control over control."

3 Summary of Ecclesiastes

The book opens up with "The words of Koheleth, son of David, King of Jerusalem," (I. 2–11), implying the book emanates from none other than Solomon.[1] This literary device gives the book a respectability that it was written by Solomon, or at least has the feel of having been written by this wisest of wise men. In fact, these words are probably written by the narrator who begins and ends the book.

Thus, there are two voices in Ecclesiastes, the narrator who frames the poem/book, and Koheleth's thoughts. According to Gordis (1951), Koheleth was probably delivering a lecture of a sort to a group of male students who had some aspirations to function in the royal court.[2]

The book begins with the famous line:

> Vanity of vanities, says Koheleth, vanity of vanities, all is vanity. What profit has a man from all his toil beneath the sun? One generation goes and another comes, but the earth is forever unchanged. The sun rises and the sun sets, breathlessly rushing towards the place where it is to rise again. Going to the south and circling to the north, the wind goes round and round, and then returns upon its tracks. All the rivers flow into the sea, but the sea is never full; to the place where the rivers flow, there they continue to flow. All things are tiresome, one cannot put them into words, and so the eye is never satisfied with seeing nor the ear filled. . . . There is nothing new under the sun.
>
> (Gordis, 1951, p. 136, I. 2–11)

Koheleth is here describing the ebb and flow of nature, a constituent part of an eternal cycle. As Perry (1993) notes, there is here a natural determinism and pessimism, namely, the concept of cyclicality such that following decline and death, there is a new start. Or to put differently, what seems to be new is actually due to the fact that the past is quickly forgotten (Gordis, 1951). Koheleth seems to be saying, on the one hand, that endless repetition is negative; however, the notion of cyclicality, which can be negative

DOI: 10.4324/9781003652816-3

or positive, opens the possibility of trying again. It is here that Koheleth exudes a tepid optimism, though there is a more pronounced pessimism and fatalism that pervades the book from what I can discern. As psychoanalyst Mark Solms noted, like Koheleth in my view, "Freud once stated that psychoanalysis is a basis for a very dark philosophy" (2024, p. 403). Koheleth and Freud have a similar outlook on the harshness of life. That is, as Koheleth suggests, "people must do their best to cope with life's vicissitudes, but risks can never be eliminated altogether" (Seow, 1997, p. 52). Most importantly, Koheleth says that everything is *hebel*, vanity. "He does not mean that everything is meaningless or insignificant," says Seow, "but that everything is beyond human apprehension and comprehension" (Seow, 1997, p. 59).

Koheleth never adequately resolves the contradiction to which all determinists are vulnerable. That is, Koheleth was assuming human freedom of choice in terms of the practical attitudes and conduct he was recommending, yet he claims that all is predetermined by God. I think that Koheleth was both advocating resigned submission to the order of the world yet also encouraging us not to be passive. In other words, in a limited sense, we have freedom of action as well as a choice between courses of action (Cohen, 1970).

Next, in section II, Koheleth engages in a "Twin experiment" (I. 12–11. 26), the first one being with wisdom. Wisdom in this context means "skill and know-how" (Heim, 2019, p. 47). More generally, wisdom refers to a deep comprehension of life's transitory nature, mindful that worldly pursuits offer no enduring satisfaction, and therefore finding meaning in living a balanced life with an emphasis on God's will, rather than only chasing material gains or earthly accomplishments. It's about perceiving the bigger picture and acceding to the limitations of human knowledge while finding satisfaction, if not contentment, in the present moment.

Koheleth's experiment with wisdom leads him to the conclusion that the search for truth in an absolute sense is pointless. Rather, God operates according to what appears to humans as an arbitrary and absolute determinism (i.e., the world is arbitrary, humans have no control, and it is unintelligible (Seow, 1997)). God does not reveal the secret as it were of existence (the mystery of divine action, (Seow, 1997)) and is thus geared to making people feel that life is often characterized by sham, drudgery, and broken dreams:

> I applied my mind to search out and explore in my wisdom all that happens beneath the sky – a sorry business it is that God has given men to be afflicted with. I have seen all the works that are done under the sun and behold all is vanity and chasing of wind, a crookedness not to be straightened, a void not to be filled.
>
> (Gordis, 1951, p. 138, I. 12-II. 26)

Koheleth then considers physical pleasure, that is, to the joys that affluence can bring, such as roomy gardens and sumptuous mansions "staffed with servants and the eternal triad of wine, women and song" (Gordis, 1951, p. 138–139):

> Then I said to myself, "Come, let me try you out in joy and enjoy pleasure," but this, too, was vanity. Of laughter I said, "It is folly," and of joy, "What good is it? . . . Whatever my eyes desired, I did not deny them; I did not deprive myself of any pleasure – for my soul rejoiced in all my labour, and that was my reward for all my labour."
>
> (Gordis, 1951, pp. 138, 140, I. 12-II. 26)

Koheleth finds the aforementioned pleasures to be gratifying for a short time, but they soon lose their thrill. He then realizes that pleasure is no more gratifying than wisdom as a reachable goal. Koheleth concludes that whatever the material pleasures he has experienced, like the fool, he ends up in the same place, namely, dead. Moreover, he concludes that whether one works hard or is lazy, the same endpoint awaits the person, termination of existence. Koheleth goes even further; to make matters worse, when he dies, after a lifetime of toil and work, some stranger, whom he may not even be acquainted with (even an offspring is in some sense a stranger), inherits his assets. Said Koheleth:

> I then turned to observe all the work that my hands had done, and all the labour I had strained to perform and lo, everything was vanity and chasing of wind, with no advantage under the sun.
>
> (Gordis, 1951, p. 140, I. 12-II. 26)

Finally, Koheleth concludes that given the aforementioned dismal constraints on living a flourishing life, the only wise goal is to strive for "joy" even though it is not an absolute belief and value. That is, it is context-dependent and setting specific:

> There is no greater good for man than eating and drinking and giving himself joy in his labour. Indeed, I have seen that this is from the hand of God, for who can enjoy a pleasure or abstain, except it be by His Will? To the man God favours He gives wisdom, knowledge and joy, but to the "sinner" He assigns the task of fathering and amassing, only to hand it over at last to the man who is pleasing to God. Indeed, this is vanity and chasing of wind.
>
> (Gordis, 1951, p. 142, I. 12-II. 26)

Section III contains the famous "Catalogue of Times" (III. 1–15). In this beautiful poetic section Koheleth alleges that all man's action is similar to events in nature, namely, they are preordained or predetermined by God. Thus, in a certain sense, all of man's actions are pointless including the quest for ultimate truth which God has concealed from men and women. Said Koheleth:

> Everything has its appointed time, and there is a season for every event under the sky.
>
> There is a time to be born, and a time to die,
> A time to plant and a time to uproot,
> A time to kill and a time to heal,
> A time to wreck and a time to build
> A time to weep and a time to laugh
> A time to mourn and a time to dance
> A time to scatter stones and a time to gather them,
> A time to embrace and a time to hold off embraces,
> A time to seek and a time to give up,
> A time to keep and a time to cast off,
> A time to tear and a time to repair,
> A time to be silent and a time to speak,
> A time to love and a time to hate,
> A time of war and a time of peace.
>
> What profit then has the worker in his toil?
> (Gordis, 1951, p. 144, III. 1–15)

Thus, as Fox (1999) notes, Koheleth is saying that every event and deed has its right or proper time, a totality of circumstances in which they should happen or be performed, and God ultimately determines when this is. However, we don't know when this context-dependent and setting-specific time is. Individuals therefore "should wait until the time is ripe rather than straining and pushing against the grain" (p. 192).

The aforementioned focus on the proper time for action in life calls to mind the Taoist notion of *wu-wei*, inaction. Wu-wei, says Watson (1968), "is not a forced quietude, but rather the renunciation of any action that is occasioned by conventional concepts of purpose or achievement, or aimed at the realization of conventional goals" (p. 468). Wu-wei, in other words, does not mean taking no action, but rather means doing nothing that is not natural or spontaneous. To the extent that one makes conscious striving and deliberate acting one's primary mode of being-in-the-world, one is bound to come in conflict with the Tao (the source of the universe that governs all things). According to Liu (1990, pp. 243, 282), there are several gradations and meanings of wu-wei in Taoist thought: wu-wei as doing nothing; wu-wei as taking as little action as possible; wu-wei as acting naturally; wu-wei as a principle of restraint, of respecting limits, especially on individual and collective narcissism, grandiosity and omnipotence. In other words, wu-wei is an attitude of care and respect for the autonomy of other things; it is selfless action.

Koheleth concludes this section of his free associations by affirming his core belief and value, namely, "I know that there is no other good in life but to be happy while one lives. Indeed, every man who eats, drinks and enjoys happiness in his work – that is the gift from God" (Gordis, 1951, p. 146, III. I-15). As I have said, following Freud, the quest for happiness is what is most important in man's doings, and for Koheleth, this means engaging the "simple" pleasures in life with the fullness of one's whole being.

In section IV (III. 16-IV. 3), Koheleth takes up the fact that "There is no justice," in discerning the way the world works:

> Furthermore, I saw under the sun that in the place of judgment there was wickedness, and in the place of righteousness, wrong. I said to myself, "Both the righteous and the wicked, God will judge, for there is a proper time for everything and every deed – over there!"
>
> (Gordis, 1951, p. 148, III. 16-IV. 3)

In other words, Koheleth was deeply troubled by the wickedness that appeared to pervade the world, including the fact that good people are subjugated by tyrants and the like. Without a strong and comforting belief in a heavenly world, man is condemned to endure his ordeal of suffering without any, or few, emotional shock absorbers. Koheleth's antidote of a type is a retreat to his core belief and value, namely, the quest for personal happiness. Such a valuative attachment, meager as it seems, appears to be the only antidote of a sort, for dealing with the harshness, or worse, of the world: "So I saw that there is nothing better for man than to rejoice in his works, for that is his lot, and no one can permit him to see what shall be afterwards" (Gordis, 1951, p. 148, III. 16-IV. 3).

Section V discusses "the folly of hard work" (IV. 4–16). That is, Koheleth opines on three reasons typically put forth for making the effort to accomplish something of lasting value. All three rationalizations are found unsatisfactory. First is the so-called joy of creation: "I saw that all hard work and skill are merely one man's rivalry with his neighbor. This too, is vanity and chasing of wind" (Gordis, 1951, p. 150). In other words, the joy of creation is driven by a wish to beat out other people, an example of the competitive urge motivating one's behavior. Put differently, Koheleth is here claiming that one might as well be lazy or under-functioning than be governed by the wish to outdo others: "But I declare: 'Better a handful acquired with ease than two hands full gained through toil and chasing after wind'" (Gordis, 1951, p. 150).

Next, Koheleth critically evaluates, with a degree of sarcasm,[3] the benefits of having a good family life, which he describes in physical terms, this being a weak foundation or justification for engaging in hard work:

> Two are better than one, because they have a reward in their labour. True, for if either falls, the other can lift his comrade, but woe to him who is

> alone when he falls, with no one else to lift him. Then also, if two sleep together, they will be warm but how can one alone keep warm?
>
> (Gordis, 1951, p. 150)

Lastly, Koheleth takes up a key narcissistic motivation for hard work which he finds unpersuasive, namely, the wish to be successful and be famous. Koheleth indicates that success and fame are passing phenomena, and it is this transitoriness that renders the quest pointless or at least dubious. Said Koheleth:

> Better a lad of poor birth, who is wise, than an old king, who is a fool and can no longer take care of himself.
>
> (Gordis, 1951, p. 152)

In Freud's famous essay *On Transience*, rather than view transience as intimidating and demoralizing, he viewed it as facilitating great value and beauty to life.

Section VI focuses "on religious etiquette" (IV. 17-V. 6), that is, the nature of piety. Koheleth is not a passionate believer, though like most Jews of that time, the temple is part of his everyday life. He thus can be described as a religious Jew of a sort. He notes as follows:

> Watch your step when you go to the house of God, for it is better to understand than to offer sacrifice like the fools, who do not even know how to do evil! Do not hasten to speak, nor let yourself be rushed into uttering words before God, for God is in heaven and you are on the earth – therefore, let your words be few.
>
> (Gordis, 1951, p. 154)

Koheleth is advocating doing one's religious obligations in the temple. He is not particularly fervent or prone to mystical ecstasy. "With all the dreams, follies and idle chatter, this remains – fear God" (Gordis, 1951, p. 154). "Fear God" roughly means "obedient gratitude" (Loader, 1986, p. 136).[4] It means to have a profound reverence, respect, and awe for God's power and authority, fundamentally acknowledging His greatness and succumbing to His will, rather than being literally fearful of Him. As Seow notes, "Despite the apparent lack of order in the world and inconsistencies of life, humankind must live in knowledge of its place in relation to the deity. This is, indeed, what Qohelet means by the 'fear of God'" (1997, p. 57).

In Section VII, "On the political scene" (V. 7, 8), Koheleth characterizes most governmental authorities as corrupt and dishonest, using its bureaucratic and hierarchical power to take advantage of the average person, especially the poor:

> If you observe the despoiling of the poor and the perversion of justice and right in the State, do not be astonished at the fact, for each guardian of the law is higher than the next, and there are still higher ones above them!
>
> (Gordis, 1951, p. 156)

Thus, Koheleth appears to have a high degree of cynicism when it comes to government, which almost always undermines a person's autonomy, integration, and humanity.

Section VIII, "The senselessness of greed," (V. 9-VI. 9). Said Koheleth:

> He who loves money will never have enough of it and he who loves wealth will never attain it – this is indeed vanity. . . . This, too, is a crying evil – as he came [into the world with nothing] so will he depart, hence what advantage was there in laboring for the wind? All his days he eats in the dark and suffers much grief, sickness and anger.
>
> (Gordis, 1951, p. 158)

Koheleth provides many of the reasons that the obsessive quest for money and wealth is vanity. The belief that having more money equates to success, happiness, and social status can motivate the obsession. Psychological factors such as perfectionism, a need for control, or low self-esteem can also contribute to an obsession with money. Koheleth would probably agree with the Apostle Paul, who famously said in the Christian Bible (1 Timothy 6:10), "For the love of money is the root of all kinds of evil."

Koheleth in particular notes that people have denied themselves many pleasures, such as hoarding their wealth for the future, only to then lose their fortune in some ill-conceived, ill-advised, and ill-fated happening, leaving their family penniless. As I said earlier, accumulated wealth, which required much personal sacrifice, is ultimately left to a stranger or one's offspring; the latter are in some sense strangers from Koheleth's point of view.

In the last entry in this section, Koheleth notes that it is God's will that men and women find/create joy in their everyday living before he dies. However, he perceptively indicates that "diligence and thrift," two of the valuative attachments of many people, are largely motivated by greed (Gordis, 1951, p. 159). For Koheleth greed means an insatiable desire for more and a sin of selfishness or pathological narcissism that can lead to emptiness and dissatisfaction:

> What advantage then has a wise man over a fool, or a poor man, who knows how to meet the problems of life? Better a joy at hand than longing for distant pleasures – that, too, is vanity and chasing of wind.
>
> (Gordis, 1951, p. 160)

In section IX, "On man's ignorance" (VI. 10–12), Koheleth repeats one of his "core" notions, namely, that events have been preordained, leaving us humans in a helpless, hopeless, and hapless state of mind. That is, there is no absolute way of discerning the meaning of life, nor is there an absolute way of predicting or even affecting the outcome of occurrences:

> What has been has already been determined, and it is known that man cannot argue with One mightier than himself. Many words merely add to

> the futility – what advantage does man derive from it? Who knows what is good for man in life, during the brief days of his vain existence, which he spends like a shadow? Who can tell man what will happen under the sun after he is gone?
>
> (Gordis, 1951, p. 162)

Koheleth is thus raising the important question, the predetermined aspect of happenings and man's helplessness before "the mystery of the world" (Gordis, 1951, p. 163).

Section X, "Thoughts on the good life" (VII. 1–14), Koheleth provides a collection of sayings that depict what he believes are the most effective attitudes for living a flourishing life. While God does not reveal what is good in any absolute sense, Koheleth takes common proverbs and gives his unique epistemological spin on them. In other words, he does not so much create new aphorisms or proverbs but uses such conventional wisdom in his idiosyncratic personal way (Fox, 2004). For example:

> Better a good name than good oil, and so the day of death rather than the day of one's birth.
>
> Better to go to a house of mourning that to a banquet-hall, for that is the end of all men and the living may take the lesson to heart.
>
> Better sorrow than laughter, for through sadness of countenance the understanding improves. Therefore, wise men prefer the house of mourning and fools the house of joy.
>
> (Gordis, 1951, p. 164)

And the last entry to this section:

> Observe the work of God, for who can straighten out what He has make crooked? In the day of good fortune enjoy it, and in the day of trouble consider that God has set the one against the other, so that man may not discover anything that happens after he is gone.
>
> (Gordis, 1951, p. 166)

In this section, Koheleth makes the important point that there are at least two ways of getting what one wants in this world, you can try and get it from others, or you can scale down your expectations. Indeed, Koheleth is suggesting that the greater the correlation between one's expectations and fate, the happier one tends to be. However, expectations are not valid predictors of experience.

In section XI, "The 'Golden Mean,'" (VIII. 15–25), Koheleth draws from the Greek wisdom of Aristotle, though some scholars reject the notion that Koheleth was influenced in any meaningful way by the Greek wisdom thinkers of the time.

In contrast, for example, Fox (1999) believes as do I, that Koheleth was influenced by Epicureanism and Stoicism, and Bartholomew (2009) makes a strong case that Koheleth was attracted by tenets of Greek thought like the autonomy of individual reason. Alter (2010), too, notes that Kohelet probably "indirectly picked up some motifs of Greek thought" (p. 338). The phrase "golden mean" is most commonly attributed to the ancient Greek philosopher Aristotle, who applied it to denote the notion of finding a virtuous middle ground between two extremes in ethics. Koheleth makes the important point that one should not strive for either extreme, saintliness or wickedness, for they both truncate a person's quest for a modicum of happiness. Says Koheleth:

> I have seen everything during my vain existence, a righteous man being destroyed for all his righteousness and a sinner living long for his wickedness. Hence do not be righteous overmuch nor be overzealous for wisdom – why be left desolate? Neither be overly wicked, nor be a fool – why die before your time? Far better to grasp the one and hold fast to the other, for he who reverences God will do his duty by both!
>
> (Gordis, 1951, p. 168)

In Koheleth, being a fool, or folly, refers to being ensconced in "material pleasures which have been prejudged as foolish . . . but not to a particular type of pleasure that is more foolish than others, because no subgroup of pleasures has been singled out" (Fox, 1999, p. 179). Folly is roughly equivalent to wickedness. "Reverences God" means to demonstrate profound respect, awe, and admiration towards God, in effect affirming His supreme power and authority while living a life correlated with His commandments, being mindful that everything emanates from Him and thus should be treated with reverence. This is often described as "fearing God" and is often regarded as the core message of the book, particularly in the concluding verse (12:13), where it states, "Fear God and keep His commandments, for that is man's whole duty" (though this was probably written by an editor or the narrator of the poem) (Gordis, 1951, p. 190).

In section XII, "On women," (VII. 26–29), Koheleth describes women in ways that suggest that he does not trust them, reflecting the prejudice of the time:

> I find woman more bitter than death, for her heart is full of traps and snares, her hands are chains. He who is favoured by God will escape her, but the sinner will be trapped by her. . . . This, too, I sought in vain, one man in a thousand I did find, but one woman among as many I could not find.
>
> (Gordis, 1951, p. 170)

Koheleth, a man of the times, appears to have some common prejudices and hang-ups regarding women, seeing them as controlling, if not castrating.

However, he also sees women as the basis of lasting happiness: "Enjoy life with the woman whom you love" (Gordis, 1951, p. 178). This entry is another example of Koheleth maintaining two contradictory perspectives.

Section XII, "Loyalty to the king" (viii. 1–9), presents Koheleth's advice to those men he was probably training for the royal court, a court that could be tyrannical and infused with intrigue, requiring adept navigating and management:

> I say: Keep the king's command, because of the oath of loyalty. Do not hasten to leave his presence but do not persist in a matter distasteful to him, for he can do whatever he wishes. Since the king's word is law, who can say to him, "What are you doing?" He who keeps his command will experience no trouble, for a wise mind will know the proper time and procedure. . . . Indeed, man does not know what the future will be, for when it happens, who will tell him?
>
> (Gordis, 1951, p. 172)

Koheleth is here giving advice on how to survive the royal court, often requiring the art of maneuvering if not manipulating, as well as skillful situational awareness. Situational awareness means having the aptitude to perceive, comprehend, and effectively react to one's circumstances. It involves understanding a given condition, gathering pertinent information, analyzing it, and making knowledgeable decisions to successfully tackle any possible risks, dangers, or events that might happen.

This being said, Koheleth is offering his sound advice based on his experience though he understands how the royal court "hangs together" and what it demands to survive there, if not flourish. He offers "tongue in cheek," good advice: a sensible underling will obey the royal court, fine tuning his responses so they are in sync with the main thrust of the king's wishes. In other words, a man should be faithful to his king because he has intimidating power that can rub him out in a moment. In fact, this calls to mind one of the reasons for Koheleth's pensive sadness, ultimately, "man is powerless over the spirit," and he "does not know what the future will be" (Gordis, 1951, p. 172).

In section XIV, "On the failure of retribution" (VIII. 10-IX. 3), Koheleth discusses the issue of reward and punishment; in this case the punishment emanates from God:

> I have seen wrong-doers being carried with pomp to their graves, and, as men return from the sacred ground, the evil-doers are praised in the city where they had acted thus. Indeed, this is vanity! . . . Here is the vanity that takes place on the earth – there are righteous men who received the recompense due to the wicked, and wicked men who receive recompense due to the righteous. I say, this is indeed vanity.
>
> (Gordis, 1951, p. 174)

Koheleth presents a rather skeptical view of "retribution" (a doctrine of merit) suggesting that in this earthly life, good deeds do not always result in positive consequences, and evil actions are not always met with just punishment, essentially questioning the idea of a clear, immediate divine justice where people receive what they deserve in this world. Moreover, sometimes punishment is exacted after an extended delay or not at all. These considerations often depict a seemingly random and unfair distribution of fortune, where both the righteous and wicked can experience similar outcomes. Koheleth thus concludes that justice is as futile as the quest for ultimate truth. Bearing in mind the aforementioned, Koheleth says:

> Therefore I praise joy, for there is no other good for man under the sun but to eat, drink, and be joyful and have this accompany him in his toil, during the days of his life, which God has given beneath the sun. . . . This is the root of the evil in all that happens under the sun – that one fate comes to all [death that is]. Therefore men's minds are filled with evil and there is madness in their hearts while they live, for they know that afterwards – they are off to the dead!
>
> (Gordis, 1951, p. 174)

In section XV, "In praise of life" (IX. 4–12), Kohelet's attitude of life-affirmation is evident: "He who is attached to all the living still has hope, for surely a live dog is better than a dead lion" (Gordis, 1951, p. 178). His sensible advice in the face of the outrageousness of life is straightforward:

> Go, then, eat your bread with joy,
> And drink your wine with a glad heart,
> For God has already approved your actions.
> At all times let your clothes be white,
> And oil on your head not be lacking.

And finally:

> Enjoy life with the woman whom you love,
> Through all the vain days of your life,
> Which God has given you under the sun
> Throughout your brief days,
> For that is your reward in life
> For your toil under the sun
>
> (Gordis, 1951, p. 178)[5]

Kohelet is here affirming the goodness of living, despite the harshness, if not pain, that seems to accompany so much of what we humans do. Moreover, he is putting into sharp focus the meaning of death anxiety, namely, death is portrayed as certain, final, and a reminder to live life to the fullest. Living well is a way of defying death, at least temporarily, and honoring a transcendent God.

Section XVI, "The inadequacies of wisdom" (IX. 13-X. 1), focuses on the problematic nature of wisdom, this being the main way to give life a sense of meaning and purpose. Koheleth's main criticisms of wisdom here is that if one lacks social status, one either does not recognize the poor man's wisdom or it is not remembered with the freshness of detail:

> So I said, "Wisdom is better than strength," but the poor man's wisdom is despised and his words go unheeded. . . . "Wisdom is better than weapons"; but I say, "One fool can destroy much good," and "As dying flies befoul the perfumer's ointment, so a little folly can outweigh an abundance of wisdom."
>
> (Gordis, 1951, p. 180)

Thus, Koheleth questions wisdom's value and that it can't guarantee a good or flourishing life. He claims that ordinary people should accept that life is unpredictable, if not random, and enjoy the simple things that come your way, or God gives you. To some extent, says Loader (1986), success depends less on skill or wisdom, "but on the unpredictable and whimsical appointments of God" (p. 112).

In section XVII, "The virtues that make for success" (X. 2-XI. 6), Koheleth provides a disconnected group of maxims that call to mind the proverbs associated with the Wisdom academies.[6] He, for example, cautions against foolishness ("A wise man's mind is his support, a fool's mind is his misfortune"); plotting to injure one's neighbor; laziness ("Through sloth the ceiling sinks, and through slack hands the house leaks"); excess in food and drink ("Send your bread upon the waters, so that you may find it again after many days"). As Gordis notes, "such virtues as prudence, energy and loyalty to the government is inculcated," and Koheleth advises his reader to diversify his business undertakings and work energetically at his appointed task, without standing idly by, to watch for wind and rain (Gordis, 1951, p. 182). Finally, Koheleth again indicates that man does not have control over his destiny; he can never discern when bad things will happen and what they may be. In other words, Koheleth's epistemiphilic drive, the drive to know, is forever stymied. However, he displays a vigilant calmness in the face of radical uncertainty, with that which is not known. This is to be contrasted with the narcissistic form of seeking, characterized by omnipotence, a kind of delusional overconfidence (Solms, 2024).

In the section XVIII, "Joy- the divine imperative" (XI. 7-XII. 8), Koheleth reasserts that it is one's duty to be happy for it is God's command to do so. Moreover, it is during one's youth when we are most alive and enlivening, that we should embrace life without reserve, for as one gets older, one becomes ill, loses one's abilities, and dies. Indeed, Koheleth says the following:

> Rejoice, young man, in your youth,
> And let your heart cheer you to your youthful days.
> Follow the impulses of your heart
> And the desires of your eyes,
> And know that for all this,
> God will call you to account.
>
> (Gordis, 1951, p. 186)

This chapter closes with the famous Allegory on Old Age, a beautiful depiction of the ageing process from the perspective of the body in decline and deterioration[7]:

> Remember your Creator in the days of your youth.
> Before the evil days come and the years draw near,
> Of which you will say, "I have no pleasure in them."
> Before the sun [the forehead] grows dark,
> And the light [the nose] of the moon [the soul] and the stars [the cheeks],
> And the clouds return after the rain [enfeebled eyesight due to trouble and sickness]
>
> In the day when watchman of the house [the flanks, ribs, arms] tremble,
> And the strong men [the legs]are bent.
> The grinding maidens [the teeth] cease, for they are few,
> And the ladies peering through the lattices [the eyes] grow dim.
>
> When the double doors on the street [ears] are shut,
> And the voice of the mill [a failing stomach] becomes low.
> One wakes at the sound of a bird,
> And all the daughters of song are laid low.

And Koheleth concludes as one gets closer to death:

> When one fears to climb a height,
> And terror lurk in a walk.
> When the almond-tree blossoms [the whitening of the hair],
> The grasshopper becomes a burden [the decline of sexual virility].
> And the cranberry [a sensual fruit] can no longer stimulate desire.
> So man goes to his eternal home, While the hired mourners walk about in the street . . .

> Before the silver cord [the tongue or the spine] is severed,
> And the golden bowl [the marrow of the head] is shattered.
> The pitcher [the gall or the stomach] is broken at the spring,
> And the wheel [skull] is shattered at the pit.
> The dust returns to the earth as it was,
> And the spirit returns to God, who gave it.
> Vanities of vanities, says Koheleth, all is vanity.
>
> (Gordis, 1951, pp. 186, 188)

The Allegory of Old Age has been interpreted in many ways. I choose to regard it as a magisterial allegory of the body in decline, as indicated previously.[8]

Koheleth presents a poignant and realistic portrayal of old age, focusing on its physical decline, loss of vitality, and the inevitability of death. It serves as a stark reminder to live life meaningfully and to remember God during youth, as the body's strength and vigor diminish with age. Overall, Koheleth's perspective on old age is a clearheaded but ultimately hopeful one. It recognizes the physical and emotional trials of aging, while at the same time reminding us of the significance of living a life that reveres God and finds/creates meaning as it confronts mortality saliency.

Section XIX, "Epilogue," (XII. 9–14), was probably written by an editor, who was both enamored with Koheleth's poetic perceptiveness, but unsettled by its radical content. Chances are this editor knew Koheleth, perhaps a fellow wisdom writer, but what is likely is that he was agitated by the subverting words that tended to undermine the traditional faith in an omnipotent, omniscient, omnipresent, and most importantly, all-good God. The last two verses of this magnificent poem[9] reflect the editors' narrative smoothing to make the entire book to be more religiously tolerable:

> Furthermore, my son, be warned: of making many books there is no end, and much study wears one's strength away
>
> In sum, having heard everything, fear God and keep His commandments, for that is man's whole duty. For God will bring every deed to judgment, even everything hidden, whether it be good or evil.
>
> (Gordis, 1951, p. 190)

Notes

1 I have liberally drawn from Gordis (1951) in this chapter.
2 What royal court, though? If the book is from the third century, there is no king of Judah, only the absentee king Ptolemy in Egypt, who occupies Judah with soldiers (Heim, personal communication).
3 Koheleth displaying this quality of sarcasm is a minority view among scholars (Heim, personal communication).

4 Gratitude is an extremely important emotion in terms of the art of living a "good life." As Sachs (2025a) points out, the famous Nun study (Snowdon, 2002) demonstrated that the more positive emotions, such as gratitude, contentment, happiness, love, and hope, the nuns expressed in their autobiographical notes in their twenties, the more likely they were to be alive and well 60 years later. The difference was as much as seven years in life expectancy. Gratitude improves physical health and immunity against disease. Grateful people are more likely to take regular exercise and go for regular medical check-ups. Thankfulness reduces toxic emotions such as resentment, frustration and regret and makes depression less likely. Gratitude, says Sachs, helps people avoid overreacting to negative experiences by seeking revenge. It even tends to make people sleep better. It enhances self-respect, making it less like that you will envy others for their achievements or success. Grateful people also tend to have better relationships. Saying "thank you" enhances friendships and potentiates better performance from employees. It is also a major factor in strengthening resilience.
5 This and the other sections who commend the pursuit of happiness through the simple things in life are often discussed as a group by biblical scholars, under the title "carpe diem" (Heim, personal communication).
6 Their existence is debated among scholars (Heim, personal communication).
7 While this is the majority view, some scholars believe it is asserted on quite shaky grounds. It is worth mentioning that there is an alternative interpretation, for example (Heim, 2019).
8 There have been many interpretations of this allegory based on Talmudic and other sources. I have mainly drawn from Cohen's (1970) *The Five Megillot* and Ginsberg's (1969) *The Five Megillot and Jonah* for my parenthetical entries. According to Heim (2019), other interpretations include, for example, the situation of an oncoming storm, household in mourning, or a judgement of God.
9 Most scholars see 1:4–11; 3:1–8, and 12:1–7 as "poems," while the rest of the book is an elevated form of writing, possibly influenced by rhetorical finesse to facilitate public performance (Heim, personal communication).

4 The Futility of Wisdom

Hokhmah, wisdom, is a key notion in Koheleth. It includes "knowledge, reasoning powers, crafts, and expertise of all sorts" (Fox, 2004, p. xx). Wisdom, in other words, is focused on "the correct ordering of life" (Loader, 1986, p. 4). In Ecclesiastes wisdom "is a practical and intellectual faculty," one that is *not* intrinsically ethical (Fox, 2004, p. xx).[1] Wisdom is a unique way of knowing, an epistemological perspective on life (Solomon et al., 2005). Koheleth uses the word *wisdom* 52 times (Murphy, 1992, p. lxi). Perhaps a rough psychoanalytic equivalent term is *ego*, the conscious part of the personality that makes decisions, calibrates the needs of the id (innate instinctive impulses) and superego (moral compass), and is governed by the reality principle (thought and action that are in sync with reality). Ego development can be comprehended as the emergence, over time, of typical ways individuals tackle differences between the features of themselves that are controllable and those features of the self that affect the person. The highest form of ego development is when a person is able to integrate numerous features of the self into a coherent narrative of self-identity, and to treasure individuality in self and others (Richardson and Pasupathi, 2005).

Somewhat differently, wisdom has been recently defined by professor of graduate education Don Ambrose as "the ability and willingness to guide one's actions through knowledge, deep understanding, fairness, altruism, and the disposition to transcend the self in order to work for the greater good" (2022, p. 258). Likewise, Sternberg and Gluck have defined wisdom as "the seeking of a common good, by achieving some balance within the person and also some balance of interests external to the person." This involves the deployment of tacit knowledge as arbitrated by values towards the objective of attaining a common good (2022, p. 12). By these definitions, Koheleth is *not* wise, though he appears to be moving in this direction. That is, Koheleth tends to be wrapped up in himself, in a self-referential personal world (Kupperman, 2005), and gives little attention to prosocial considerations. Instead, he seems to be lodged in the norm of reciprocity, "I do for you and you do for me." In fact, as H.L. Ginsberg (1969) notes, Koheleth "recommends generosity with a purely utilitarian motivation (one will then be more likely to be

DOI: 10.4324/9781003652816-4

shown generosity if one should ever need it)" (p. 55). In contrast, Seow (1997) believes that Koheleth's "chief concerns are with the plight of humanity and with the quest for what is good for humanity" (p. 67).

While there is no consensus in the psychological literature about what in fact wisdom is, based on a literature review and consensus opinion of a panel of experts, wisdom has been defined as a multifaceted trait involving balanced integration of nine elements (Carr, 2022, p. 222): (1) Expert social decision-making ability and pragmatic knowledge of life (Koheleth appears in part to be rather befuddled, if not troubled by life). (2) Prosocial attitudes and behavior (Koheleth shows little regard for the best interests of others, on their own terms). (3) A capacity to maintain emotional homeostasis with a bias towards positive emotions (Kohelelth lacks emotional homeostasis, he is rather labile and has a bias towards negative emotions). (4) A capacity for reflection and understanding (Koheleth shows this capacity to a fault, though he tends to be self-referential). (5) A capacity to expect and cope with uncertainty (Koheleth appears to be deeply worried at the uncertainty in life and the lack of control that it implies). (6) Tolerance for different values in others and an understanding of the relativity of values (Koheleth appears to have these qualities). (7) Spirituality (Koheleth is not a particularly spiritual person, though he does believe in God). (8) Openness to new experiences (Koheleth is open to new experience, in fact he unsuccessfully tries just about everything to make himself feel better). (9) A sense of humor (Koheleth, says Heim (2019), is a humorous character, a tragicomic one that is).

Koheleth's main claim is that wisdom, the "means" that Koheleth applies to investigate life as well as its goal (Fox, 1999, p. 172), has not provided him with the basis for a meaningful, satisfying, or transcendent life. In fact, wisdom has failed him as a tool for unraveling the mystery of the world (e.g., the inscrutable God) and effectively navigating his own existential odyssey. All is *hevel* (futility*)*.[2]

As Perry (1993) notes, Koheleth is a "*homme absurd*" (p. 16), a concept that Crenshaw (1987, p. 23) also uses in his commentary: "Life is profitless; totally absurd," as does Fox (1999). Following French philosopher Albert Camus, the three possible responses to the absurd in traditional absurdism are **revolt,** that is, living life with passion and freedom, despite the futility or senselessness of life. Koheleth comes across as an impassioned thinker, one whose freedom is manifested mainly as attitudinal freedom despite the absurdity of life. As with the Stoics (and Freud), Koheleth emphasizes accepting reality, living in the present, and focusing on what you can control. **Acceptance,** that is, accepting the absurd condition and living in defiance of it. Indeed, throughout his book, Koheleth notes the absurdity to ordinary life, but defies its hold on him by his ultimately embracing life without reserve (i.e., enjoying the "blessings" that comes his way, since man is ignorant of what lies ahead (Fox, 1999)) and fearing God and keeping his commandments (i.e., revering and obeying God by living a righteous life).[3] Fearing God means respecting "the distance between the divine and the human" (Seow, 1997, p. 201). Finally, **rejection of escape**, that is, rejecting suicide and help from a higher power (e.g., God.) Suicide and denial were not options for Koheleth because they were types of escapism and deceiving oneself. Koheleth never considers suicide though he does say that it was better to have not been born than live in the absurd world as he perceives it, a view that recapitulates what is written in the Talmud on this subject.[4] He also does not give God a major redemptive role in his discourse (though God is viewed as the Creator of all things and one should be obedient to Him). Likewise, Koheleth comes across as dedicated truth-teller, including the tough truths that constitute authentic living as he conceives it.

While Koheleth does not make a pronounced distinction between wisdom and knowledge, it seems that this is an important omission. Briefly, knowledge can be defined as comprehending basic facts, truths, and information. It is largely an intellectualized activity (e.g., bookish knowledge, intellectual nimbleness). We obtain knowledge from learning and education. Wisdom is the ability to use knowledge in a pragmatic, smart manner.[5] Most scholars believe wisdom emanates from everyday experiences. For example, knowledge is knowing what to say, wisdom is knowing whether to say it or not. Tomatoes are a fruit, but using them in a fruit salad is ill-conceived. Knowledge always comes prior to wisdom. Wisdom is lodged in knowledge. This means that you can be both wise and knowledgeable, but you can't be wise without being knowledgeable. And just because you're knowledgeable doesn't necessarily mean you're wise.

As Carr (2022) points out, cognitive/social scientist Igor Grossman has conceptualized wisdom as an advanced stage of cognitive development characterized by what he calls "wise reasoning." Here is a summary of Grossman's theory.

Wise reasoning, says Carr, is a set of cognitive capabilities useful for solving complex, poorly defined problems that requires more than the ability for abstract reasoning and logic (i.e., knowledge). Wise reasoning involves four important competencies, competencies that Koheleth displays: (1) Intellectual humility, or knowing the limits of one's knowledge. For example, Koheleth is frustrated by him knowing that he cannot fathom God's actions or for that matter, how His world "hangs" together. He humbly, though somewhat begrudgingly, resigns himself to these constraints. (2) Recognizing that, in complex situations, there is uncertainty about the stability of people's positions and their openness to change. Koheleth is deeply troubled by the fact that there appears to be so much uncertainty that constitutes everyday life. Similar to the Stoics, he focuses on what is controllable. (3) Seeking multiple perspectives on complex problems, as single perspectives may not fully reflect all the complexities of the situation. Koheleth experiments with many social paradigms of his day finding them all wanting. (4) Finally, integrating different perspectives, sometimes through negotiation and compromise. By the end of the book, Koheleth compromises; on one hand he knows he cannot fathom the mystery of the world, or God's ways, and on the other, he somewhat begrudgingly decides to enjoy whatever blessings come his way. As the saying goes, "God writes straight with crooked lines," that is, even though life may seem chaotic, full of swings and roundabouts, and seemingly negative events, God is still working behind the scenes, as it were, to achieve a greater good, ultimately guiding our lives towards a positive path, even if we can't perceive it at the time.

Koheleth indicates in section II, "the twin experiment" (I. 12–11. 26), that wisdom has failed him:

> I, Koheleth, was king over Israel in Jerusalem [Koheleth pretends he is King Solomon]. I applied my mind to search out and explore in my wisdom all that happens beneath the sky – a sorry business it is that God has given men to be afflicted with. I have seen all the works that are done under the sun and behold all is vanity and chasing of wind, a crookedness not to be straightened, a void not to be filled.
>
> (Gordis, 1951, p. 138)

Moreover:

> Said I to myself, "Here I have greatly increased my wisdom, beyond all those who were before me over Jerusalem, for my heart has attained much wisdom and knowledge." But as I applied my mind, I learnt that wisdom and knowledge are madness[6] and folly. Yes, I perceived that this, too, is chasing after wind. For the more wisdom the more grief, and increasing one's knowledge means increasing one's pain.
>
> (Gordis, 1951, p. 138)

Koheleth concludes from the aforementioned that the quest for Truth with a capital "T" is useless and designed only to make men unhappy (Gordis, 1951). Like the anti-realist he is, Koheleth seems to believe that there is no such thing as objective truth that can be comprehended, even apprehended, and all knowledge is ultimately subjective, local, situated, and contextually bounded agreements and conventions (Osbeck and Robinson, 2005). This is one of the postmodern aspects of Ecclesiastes. That is, Koheleth appears to intuitively recognize that all evidence and facts are discourse specific, contestable, and can never be absolutely adjudicated. This self-awareness is bothersome to Koheleth.

In the section "the inadequacies of wisdom" (IX. 13-X-1), Koheleth makes the important point that in general, wisdom is hardly honored in society:

> This also I saw as an instance of wisdom under the sun, and it seemed significant to me. A small city there was, with few people in it, and a great king attacked it, besieging it and building breastworks against it. But was

> found in it a poor wise man who saved the city by his wisdom, yet no one remembered the poor man. So I said, "Wisdom is better than strength," but the poor man's wisdom is despised and his works go unheeded.
>
> (Gordis, 1951, p. 180)

In this anecdote, Koheleth is suggesting that the wise man who is poor and lowly in social status rarely receives the honor he deserves; in fact, often his counsel is ignored even though he saves the day. What also irks Koheleth is the fact that " 'one fool can destroy much good,' and 'As dying flies befoul the perfumer's ointment, so a little folly can outweigh the abundance of wisdom' " (Gordis, 1951, p. 180). In other words, one act of folly can spoil an accomplishment of wisdom.

The wise person has been described as one who "knows that one does not know" ("The only true wisdom," said Socrates, "is in knowing you know nothing"), and we fear along with Erik H. Erikson that no one who is truly wise would ever claim to be so. Perhaps the most valid attribution of wisdom must come from affirming others (Peterson and Seligman, 2004). That is, the paradox of wisdom is that someone who views himself as wise is quite likely to be overpositive, obstinate, and egoistic (Kupperman, 2005).

Fox (2004) clearly describes the main dilemma that Koheleth faces:

> The heart of the book is life's absurdities frustrate the rational mind . . . the irrationality of the world is his fundamental grievance. . . . We cannot know what will come to pass, so we must grasp whatever blessings the moment offers.
>
> (pp. xvii, xxx, 47)

Freud would probably agree with the aforementioned description of the human condition as well as its recommendation.

From a Freudian point of view, raising such meaning-oriented questions are a sign of psychological distress, if not mental illness. Said Freud in a letter to French psychoanalyst Marie Bonaparte on August 13, 1937:

> The moment a man questions the meaning and value of life, he is sick, since objectively neither has any existence; by asking this question one is merely admitting to a store of unsatisfied libido to which something else must have happened, a kind of fermentation leading to sadness and depression.
>
> (Freud, 1937/1961, pp. 436–437)

And elsewhere in *Civilization and Its Discontents*, Freud appealed directly to his naturalistic assumption, when he asserts that one has "a right to dismiss the question of the meaning of life, for it seems to derive from human presumptuousness. Nobody talks about the purpose of life of animals" (Patterson, 1984,

p. 78). And finally, in a letter to his friend and collaborator Wilhelm Fleiss, Freud felt compelled to reassert the same point: "When we begin to ask ourselves questions about the meaning of life and death, we are sick, for none of that exists objectively" (Ferry, 2005, p. 122). Of course, Freud's view on the meaning and value of life is highly debatable, as contemporary Freudian and other analysts have suggested. However, like Koheleth, Freud has a "dark" view of the human situation. He believed that life is a constant struggle between two opposite forces: the life instinct (Eros) and the death instinct (Thanatos). He also believed that man is fundamentally pleasure-seeking in an erotically tinged universe. While Koheleth speaks about love in his book, he gives skimpy comment on sexuality, for example, saying in one allegorical translation/commentary that as one gets older, one's sexual function and vitality declines ("The grasshopper becomes a burden").[7] As Freud noted in *Civilization and Its Discontents*, "The sexual life of civilized man is notwithstanding severely impaired; it sometimes gives the impression of being in process of involution as a function, just as our teeth and hair seem to be organs" (Freud, 1930, p. 105).

Koheleth's reflections take place when he is an old, thoughtful man and thus can be usefully conceptualized as occurring amidst the last psychosocial stage of personality development that psychoanalyst Erik. H. Erikson calls "Ego Integrity versus Despair." Integrity versus despair is comprised of a retrospective reflection about life and either feeling content that life was well-lived (integrity) or regretting decisions and missed opportunities (despair). As Carr (2022) points out, research on lifespan development strongly suggests that individuals do face the psychosocial dilemmas described by Erikson's theory and develop the virtues (like wisdom) or vulnerabilities (despair) associated with successful or unsuccessful resolution of them, continuously and cumulatively over the lifespan.

As Erikson notes, integrity is the result of the previous seven stages of the life cycle. It evolves in the adult whose ego can accept his life cycle "as something that had to be and that by necessity, permitted of no substitutions; it thus means a new, a different love of one's parents" (Erikson, 1950, p. 268). The adult in whom ego integrity has fully bloomed recognizes that his individual life is but one life cycle in the flow of history. He is convinced that what had to be, was, and was basically gratifying. Says Erikson on wisdom or ego-integrity: "It is the acceptance of one's own and only life cycle and of the people who have become significant to it as something had to be and that by necessity, permitted of no substitution" (Erikson, 1959, p. 98). The danger, Monte (1980) explains, is that the ego may have failed to integrate the crisis resolutions of the previous seven stages of life development. The fear of death that is in sharp focus means that the individual is unwilling and unable to accept his life cycle as the ultimate one and only meaning that living exemplifies. Despair of what has been implies that what has been, has been in vain. Despair, says Monte, is the protest of a person who is not yet satisfied with a life that has never been satisfying. Despair indicates an unwillingness, paradoxical as it may be, to end a life that has failed to accomplish satisfaction and that now culminates as the sum of a thousand little miseries. The virtue or ego strength that serves as the hallmark of the climactic stage of the life cycle is Wisdom. "Wisdom . . . is detached concern with life itself, in the face of death itself" (Erikson, 1964, p. 133), "truly involved disinvolvement" (Erikson, 1982, p. 61). Adults who embody the kind of integrity that Erikson describes are wise in the sense that they view their limited lives as a totality that transcends petty disgust at the feeling of "being finished." They are able to transcend the despair, "of facing the period of relative helplessness which makes the end as it marked the beginning" (Erikson, 1964, p. 134). With wisdom or integrity there is "an increased sense of inner unity" (Erikson, 1959, p. 51) or "a sense of coherence and wholeness" (Erikson et al., 1986, p. 65).

As psychoanalyst Salman Akhtar (2009) summarizes, this last stage of Eriksonian life cycle development, ego integrity versus despair, it encompasses many subsets of human capacities, ideally leading to wisdom. This includes the following:

1. *A post-narcissistic love of the human, not personal self.* Koheleth's outlook appears to be mainly narcissistic, that is, it is focused on his pleasure and joy rather than, or in addition to, serving the other on his own terms. For Erikson, this narcissistic outlook can be considered unwise. That is, wisdom is characterized by prosocial attitudes and behavior. Koheleth cannot be reasonably characterized as oriented to "generative wisdom, that is, particular products, outcomes, or initiatives that are geared toward enhancing the welfare of generations to come." This type of wisdom is generative in the way that Erikson says he uses the notion, "a concern in establishing and guiding the next generation" (Solomon et al., 2005, pp. 272–273).
2. *A sense of spirituality.* For Erikson, this spirituality can take on many different forms; what characterizes such spiritualities is that they are mainly self-transcending. While Koheleth has some "god-talk" in his book, for the most part, he does not find spirituality/religion to be useful in his efforts to find/create transcending meaning via wisdom. As positive psychologist Michael Levenson notes, transcendence is a developmentary trajectory that forms a pathway to wisdom. Self-transcendence is accomplished as we pass through phases of self-knowledge, detachment, and integration (Carr, 2022).
3. *An acceptance of the actuality and inevitability of one's life.* Koheleth appears to accept his dying; in fact, he sometimes claims that in certain contexts, it was better to not have been born. For the most part, Koheleth views his death as part of a monotonous natural cycle. "There is a time to be born, and a time to die" (Gordis, 1951, p. 144). As I have said, for Erikson wisdom involves the acceptance of one's own life as the best one could have lived, an acceptance of the inevitability of death. As Bartholomew has noted in his wonderful commentary of Ecclesiastes, "Any wisdom worth

its weight has to come to terms with death, the great enigma of life" (Bartholomew is quoting McIntire, 2020, p. 118). The question that one should ask oneself is, if you knew you were going to die tomorrow, how would you live today? (Gibson, 2017).

4. *A deep acceptance of the character flaws and strengths of one's parents.* There is no mention of Koheleth's parents or early upbringing in his book. According to Gordis (1951), scholars have inferred that Ecclesiastes was probably something of a country gentleman, a bachelor with no children who possibly came from a comfortable upper-middle-class background with a socially and politically conservative outlook. Zimmermann (1973), however, believes that Koheleth was in a lousy marriage and had a son.

   Since there is no information in the book whatsoever, all here is of course speculative.
5. *Pride in the dignity of one's lifestyle and what Erikson called "the patrimony of one's soul," that is, the seal of moral paternity of oneself.*

   Koheleth appears to believe that in general, his life as he has experienced it via wisdom has not been very satisfying. However, it is a sign of wisdom that he could more or less live with contradiction and paradox (Compton and Hoffman, 2020).
6. *In the absence of such accumulated wisdom, the individual keeps feeling that he or she could have lived a different life and, since no time is left to redo or undo life, experiences a deep sense of despair.* Peaceful acceptance of the coming end of one's life is replaced by a deep fear of death. Koheleth does experience his fair share of despair at the lack of effectiveness of wisdom in his existential odyssey. He views the world as being a repetitive monotonous cycle in which there is nothing new under the sun. Moreover, while he does not seem to be very afraid of dying, he also does not feel that his application of wisdom has been very useful in his living. As Freud famously noted, "If you want to endure life, prepare yourself for death" (1915, p. 300).[8] That is, mortality salience can be a basis for propulsive living not futility as Koheleth tends to view it. As psychoanalyst Ralph Kahana noted about Freud for example, he "was unusually concerned with his own mortality, and had an intense and lifelong dislike of aging, especially as it entailed any decline in his creativity." However, "in retrospect, these attitudes contrast, ironically, with his eventual longevity; his scientific and literary achievements in late life; and his courage facing a prolonged illness and death" (Kahana, 1978, p. 39).

Thus, Koheleth's outlook on wisdom and the like, at least in part, calls to mind the aforementioned description by Erikson of the psychosocial stage of ego integrity versus despair. Koheleth appears to be on-and-off in a state of despair, though he also affirms embracing pleasure and joy without reserve.

Here is a clinical vignette about a patient struggling with integrity versus despair, that calls to mind Koheleth's personal struggles:

Lauren, age 74, came to me after having been in what she described as a largely unhelpful four-times-a-week psychoanalysis that lasted over three decades. While she felt that the treatment helped her maintain her job as an executive secretary in a large law firm, she was never able to find love, that is, get married (or have a life partner) and have children. She believed that she was too "broken" to do so, and the analysis did not help her correct this perspective. She said that in hindsight, she was "addicted" to her previous therapist, whom she believed unconsciously cultivated her dependence on her.

Lauren called me, in part, because she was amidst a payment dispute with her ex-analyst who owed her many thousands of dollars but refused to pay her back (the therapist appears to have been "double dipping" around Medicare and co-pays for years), leading to her taking her analyst to court for a remedy. She prevailed in court, and she and her analyst made a settlement in which she got all of what she owed Lauren, $18,000. Lauren felt that as a result of the way the treatment ended, in a terrible money dispute, with her analyst lying to her, she claimed, she "beat herself up" over having so misjudged her analyst's character and stayed with her so many years. While her analyst helped her retain her job, she felt she was manipulated by her. This being said, Lauren felt betrayed by her analyst though she also missed her, feeling her life was spinning out of control. Coming to me three times a week was her way of getting some control over her life, which she often felt was chaotic and largely unsatisfying. Lauren indicated to me that by coming to see me she "got out of the house" and "had someone to talk to," which helped settle her. I had been seeing her for about six months. Being retired for about a decade, Lauren had some good friends whom she regularly met with, and she spent a lot of time going to movies and on short vacations alone.

In the transference, I was the "good" therapist whom she could trust, though she frequently put me down as a way of keeping her distance. I found Lauren to be very interesting and funny, though a pained woman, who was in the last phase of her challenging life. She lacked any firm basis for experiencing her life as meaningful and wanted her ordeal of suffering to end.

This being said, Lauren was in a state of despair for she had been living in a loveless hell for most of her adult life. She felt that she "missed the boat" on having a satisfying life, particularly because she never married, or had a long-term romance, nor had children. About the latter, she claimed that she would have been a terrible mother, coming from a "crazy family." I more or less agreed with her self-assessment. Lauren appeared to have difficulties being nurturing and stable. Lauren told me that she hoped to die when she was age 80, feeling there was nothing substantial to live for, and she was terrified of physical disintegration.

I should mention that Lauren had long-term shingles for about 12 years, and this condition was frequently very painful making her everyday life feel "unbearable," as she told me. A painful itchy rash was her main symptom, and she was addicted to the narcotic Percocet, a controlled substance painkiller that she received from an unscrupulous psychiatrist. I gently pointed out to Lauren that her physical pain was in part motivating her to feel that pressing forward in her life was futile for her pain might last the rest of her life. She responded by telling me that I was stating the obvious and I was a "lightweight therapist."

Lauren said that she would leave her assets to some cousins whom she felt somewhat close to. She hoped that she had the will and ability to kill herself when the time came (by Percoset and liquor). When I pointed out that Ben Franklin was age 70 when he signed the Declaration of Independence, Mother Teresa was age 87 before she retired, and Grandma Moses was 78 when she began painting, Lauren sarcastically noted that she was no Ben Franklin, Mother Teresa, or Grandma Moses. She called my analogy "one of the stupidest things" she has heard by a therapist.

As I have indicated, according to Erikson's psychosocial development theory, integrity is typified by a sense of acceptance, peace of mind, and satisfaction with one's life, often accompanied by feelings of wisdom and a lack of regret. In contrast, despair is characterized by reflecting back on one's life with feelings of regret, shame, disappointment, and a sense that life was wasted, often leading to bitterness and hopelessness. Lauren was a classic example of a person in quiet despair. In her "life review," conceived as the construction, interpretation, and evaluation of her life course (Jordan, 2005), she viewed herself as a failure, "as wasting my life." My work with her focused on helping her find/create some meaning structures that could sustain her in the time she had left, even suggesting that she try internet dating, a suggestion that she felt was "dumb" given her age and circumstance. Lauren indicated that no man (or woman) would want a "cantankerous, old crotchety woman."

For the most part, I felt that Lauren was correctly characterizing her life as one of missed opportunities, of sham, drudgery, and broken dreams. This being said, I believed that even in the mid-seventies, Lauren's life needed not be void of personal achievement and growth (Jordan, 2005). I was cautiously optimistic that I could help her a bit as she struggled through this last painful phase of her life cycle.

Conclusion

Koheleth alleges that life as a totality of circumstances is vanity, senseless, or absurd. "The point of the book as a whole," says Seow in his superb commentary, "is that all people, male and female, are under the burden of toil" (1997, p. x). He in part, views his struggles in life to be metaphorically analogous to Sisyphus, who is fated to be in Hades to forever roll a boulder uphill and only to lose it to gravity at the top of the hill and have to begin all over again, continually (McIntire, 2020). Or to put it differently, in ethical terms, "we are all born with limited capacities to pursue the good, and left to our own devices all of us betray ourselves and our fellow man" (Patterson, 1984,

p. 89). However, according to Koheleth, the last six verses, probably written by the more orthodox narrator or someone else, indicate that the partial antidote to this tragicomic outlook is as follows:

> In sum, having heard everything, fear God and keep His Commandments, for that is man's whole duty. For God will bring every deed to judgment, even everything hidden, whether it be good or evil.
>
> (Gordis, 1951, p. 190)

The idea here is that wisdom is capable of bringing life into a correlation with the divine will and purpose. In other words, perhaps the message of Koheleth is not so much when we modify the way we conceptualize God, but when it animates the way we love and serve God with the lives and love we possess. Put succinctly, the kind of meaning that can sustain one amidst the shocks of existence that must be borne to realize one's better nature is to recognize, if not affirm, that authentic meaning emanates from God. Indeed, Heim has succinctly made this point in his excellent commentary when he wrote the following:

> The main point of the entire book: the divine retribution of the emotional and material goods that his wayward audience were hoping to achieve without God renders their goals a *mirage* and *chasing after wind.* With this, the Solomonic persona has completed his didactic task, and for the remainder of the book Qoheleth abandons it and resumes his original identity as a public orator.
>
> (Heim, 2019, p. 64)

In this context then, says Heim, Koheleth does not advocate "resignation, rather, he promotes realism and fosters resilience" (2019, p. 91). Koheleth seems to be mindful that individuals can never know everything that is essential to discern the best decision in the present, to perfectly well forecast the future, or to be 100% certain about why things occurred the way they did in the past. In other words, a wise person is mindful of uncertainty and has cultivated ways to cope with it (Staudinger et al., 2005). Put differently, says Seow, "no human can tell 'what is good'" (1997, p. 251).

The possible implication of the aforementioned is that Koheleth, who appears to have a high wisdom-related knowledge, has a deep understanding of the complexity of life, especially its low points. Therefore, a wise person like Koheleth is likely to experience some level of "constructive melancholy." In other words, because Koheleth has a high level of wisdom knowledge, he probably spontaneously reacted strongly to certain basic life events because of his deep understanding of the significance of these events. Viewed over time, Koheleth's wisdom-related knowledge should bring about the down-regulation of negative emotions (e.g., pessimism, cynicism), so that he does not behave dysfunctionally (Kunzmann and Baltes, 2005).

Thus, Koheleth is probably right: Godless life under the sun renders most things ultimately pointless; however, he also alleges, correctly I believe, that if we put our faith in something else that is not under the sun, we are more likely to experience self-transcendence and the joy and gratitude it brings (Ryken, 2015).

For there is in the heart of man a wish for something more, something higher, something better. Put differently, perhaps the ultimate message of Koheleth is not that nothing matters, that there is nothing new under the sun, but rather, everything matters, and there is nothing old under the sun. Put your faith in something else that is not under the sun (Ryken, 2015), and you have a reasonable chance to find/create a way of being in the world suffused with meaning and purpose.

Notes

1 According to Heim (personal communication) this is a controversial claim.

2 According to Rabbi Jonathan Sachs, the key word *hevel*, which Gordis translates as "futility," is actually a mistranslation. *Hevel*, says Sachs, means "a fleeting breath." The book is not a study in disillusionment but rather it is about the brevity of life on earth (Sachs, 2025c).

3 Fearing God is a way of denoting terror and shrinking from Him (Loader, 1986).

4 The sages taught in the Talmud the following *baraita* (a baraita is a traditional Jewish teaching that was not included in the Mishnah, the first authoritative codification of Jewish law). For two and a half years Beit (the "house") Shammai and Beit Hillel disagreed. These say: It would have been preferable had man not been created than to have been created. And those said: It is preferable for man to have been created than he not been created. Ultimately, they were counted and concluded: It would have been preferable had man not been created than to have been created. However, now that he has been created, he should examine his actions that he has performed and seek to correct them. And some say: He should scrutinize his planned actions and evaluate whether or not and in what matter those actions should be performed, so that he will not sin. *https://www.sefaria.org ›... › Daf 13b › Line 11 Accessed 2/20/25*

5 See especially Maxwell (2007).

6 Madness for Koheleth refers to unbridled and unprincipled behavior, as a function of believing that life is vanity and that there is no moral law operating in the world (Gordis, 1951).

7 Gordis believes this is an allusion to the decline of sexual virility (1951, p. 188).

8 Freud's statement calls to mind Noble laureate Daniel Kahneman, who lived this principle until the end of his life. Kahneman, despite being relatively healthy, died by assisted suicide at age 90 in Switzerland. As Kahneman saw it, to live well, one needs to be able to ask when a life is complete (Lazari-Radek and Singer, 2025).

5 The Futility of Hedonism

Hedonism is a philosophy that emphasizes pleasure-seeking and evading pain. That is, the royal road to happiness in hedonism is the pursuit of pleasure, its maximization, while also avoiding physical and mental pain. Epicureanism is a sub species of hedonism, a philosophy that emphasizes moderation and the avoidance of extremes. The Epicureans quested after happiness, through pleasure and freedom, without fearfulness (Fox, 2004). Koheleth early on in his book, after he unsuccessfully uses wisdom to find/create happiness, immerses himself in physical and mental pleasure-seeking:

> Then I said to myself, "Come, let me try you out in joy and enjoy pleasure," but this too was vanity. Of laughter I said, "It is folly," and of joy, "What good is it?"
>
> For I explored the matter with my mind, by stimulating the body with wine (while my mind was acting with wisdom) and by taking hold of frivolity, so that I might see what course is best for men under the sky during the brief span of their lives.
>
> (Gordis, 1951, pp. 139–140, I. 12-II. 26)

Koheleth, the experimental hedonist (Ryken, 2015), also tells us that he built beautiful, spacious mansions for himself and planted luscious vineyards; he laid out gardens and parks and planted a wide range of fruit-trees; he made pools of water, to water a forest of trees; he bought both male and female slaves, though he had many slaves and a large household; he owned much cattle and sheep more than anyone else in Jerusalem; he amassed silver and gold and treasures of kings and provinces; he acquired singers; he engaged in sex with many mistresses; overall, Koheleth added to his possessions beyond all who had been before him in Jerusalem, while his wisdom remained with him.[1]

In a nutshell says Koheleth:

> Whatever my eyes desired, I did not deny them; I did not deprive myself of any pleasure – for my soul rejoiced in all my labour, and that was the reward for all my labour.
>
> (Gordis, 1951, p. 140)

DOI: 10.4324/9781003652816-5

Koheleth tells us that while he found the aforementioned pleasure-seeking satisfying in the short term, ultimately it was vanity, chasing after the wind. The reason for this meaningless hedonism appears to be satiation and the boredom and other negative emotions that usually accompanies such pleasure-seeking after the initial exhilaration. Ultimately, says Koheleth, pleasures and achievements do not endure, for everything is ephemeral (Gibson, 2017). Put differently, Koheleth is radically self-indulgent in his quest for self-centric pleasure. As Emmanuel Levinas would put it, there is almost nothing in this quest for pleasure that is other-directed, other-regarding, or other-serving.

Hedonism as an ethical lifestyle has been criticized for many reasons. For example, Immanuel Kant argued that a life dedicated only to pleasure-seeking is superficial, insubstantial and unsatisfying, while others, like John Stuart Mill claimed that hedonism can lead to self-indulgence (as with Koheleth), neglect of moral obligations, and injury to others.

The central criticisms of hedonism comprise as follows: the paradox of hedonism (questing after pleasure directly can reduce its importance, that is, limits are the essence of pleasure); the notion that not all pleasures are similarly valuable; the potential for neglecting other significant features of life like morality and meaning; and the problematic nature of accurately measuring and comparing different kinds of pleasures; fundamentally, claiming that pleasure alone cannot be the only determinant or motivation of a good or flourishing life.

While Epicureanism is considered a sub-species of hedonism, the main difference lies in its stress on questing after simple, natural pleasures and avoiding pain, rather than actively questing after intense or extravagant pleasures, which is how hedonism is usually understood; fundamentally, Epicureanism argues for a more moderate and restrained approach to pleasure seeking, prioritizing tranquility over immediate gratification of one's desires.

Fox (1999) distinguishes pleasure, happiness, and joy as the terms are used in Koheleth. He claims pleasure is not an independent emotion or sensation, but a feeling-tone connected to more comprehensive experiences. A pleasure like sex may stimulate that feeling-tone, but in certain circumstances, like a person suffering from anhedonia (inability to feel/express pleasure), one may not feel any meaningful pleasure. Pleasure, then, refers to the immediate and often physical sensation of enjoyment or satisfaction. Koheleth appears to experience a degree of pleasure as he enacts his hedonic behavior early on in his book, though it does not last very long.

This is very different from happiness. Happiness, says Fox, is an emotion, an experience that has an all-encompassing hold on consciousness while it is in play. He notes that pleasure is often, though not always, a contributing aspect to happiness. Some individuals like my patient who has a sexual addiction, feels some pleasure in her exploits, yet at the end of the experience she feels a lingering emptiness, depression, and guilt. On the other hand, some individuals, like my 77-year-old male patient who has a sexless marriage, is happy even though he lacks sexual pleasure. Happiness then, is a long-term state of tranquility and satisfaction. For the most part, Koheleth does not experience the aforementioned contentment and fulfillment. He is a very troubled soul.

Finally, says Fox, joy connotes an intense and stable kind of happiness focused on a praiseworthy object such as one's family and achievements. In the case of my patient with a sexless marriage, he says that he unambivalently loves his wife and often experiences an upsurge of joy when with her. Fundamentally then, happiness is a moment, while joy is a more sustained state of being-in-the-world.

With regards to Koheleth, it is important to clarify one other confusion, namely, that a person who is happy has necessarily found/created meaning. That is, while happiness and meaning are similar, they are not the same. For example, says Jonathan Sachs (2025b), happiness is mainly about satiating one's needs and desires. In contrast, meaning is about a sense of purpose in life, especially by making positive contributions to the lives of others. Happiness is focused on how one feels in the present while meaning is how you judge your life as a whole: past, present, and future. Finally, happiness is linked to taking while meaning is linked to giving. In a word, there can be happiness without meaning, and there can be meaning in the absence of happiness, even while suffering (Viktor Frankl's logotherapy comes to mind). As Sachs further notes, individuals who suffer are not happy, but they may be living lives rich with meaning.

By the end of his book, Koheleth appears to be devoted to joy as a superordinate belief and value. In fact, there are seven *carpe diem* passages that occur in Ecclesiastes, all of which "celebrate creaturely human life as God has made it" (Bartholomew, 2009, p. 152.). That is, despite all of the trials and tribulations, Koheleth says it is his "duty to enjoy life and taste its pleasures in full" (Gordis, 1951, p. 240). "Simple hedonism is a gift of God" (Alter, 2010, p. 364). Says Koheleth:

> Go, then, eat your bread with joy.
> And drink your wine with a glad heart,
> For God has already approved your actions.
> At all times let your clothes be white,
> And oil on your head not be lacking.
> Enjoy life with the woman who you love,
> Through the vain days of your life,
> Which God has given you under the sun,
> Throughout your brief days,
> For that is your reward in life
> For your toil under the sun.
> (Gordis, 1951, p. 178)

What Koheleth is getting at has been succinctly stated by Heim (2019): "Qoheleth concludes that *there is nothing better for humans than to take delight in all they do*. The ability to do this, however, is dependent on God" (p. 75). God in this instance is characterized by Koheleth as eternal, all-knowing, just (usually), and in ultimate control (sort of). Such a valuative attachment calls to mind a famous passage from the Babylonian Talmud: "Everyone must give an account before God of all good things one saw in life and did not enjoy" (Seow, 1997, p. 371).

In psychoanalysis, man is animated by the pleasure-unpleasure principle (referred to these days as the "pleasure principle"). This principle claims that the mind tends to avoid pain or unpleasure and pursues pleasure, probably an ancient Hedonist/ Epicurean influence on Freud's theorizing. For example, Freud regarded Epicureanism as a philosophy that shares an important core notion with his psychoanalytic theory, namely, the questing after pleasure and avoidance of pain. Freud viewed Epicureanism as an early philosophical expression of this basic human drive towards pleasure.

Unpleasure, the stronger of the two tendencies, is a consequence of the accumulation of instinctual tensions and pleasure from the discharge of this tension (Akhtar, 2009). With development and growth, the individual is moderated by the reality principle, the ego's control of the pleasure-seeking activity of the id so as to satisfy the demands of the outside world. Anxiety or any perceived danger by the ego, activates defenses, and the pleasure-unpleasure principle is operative in protecting oneself from the threat (Akhtar, 2009). In psychoanalysis, one of the goals of analysis is to embrace pleasure-seeking, though what can be called responsible pleasure seeking in which for example, as I have said, limits are the essence of pleasure-seeking.

Responsible pleasure seeking is based on the Freudian premise that man is essentially pleasure-seeking in an erotically tinted universe. In other words, Freud the hedonist believed that the seeking after pleasure is the master key to meaning in life. Happiness and the good life are conceptualized in terms of pleasure seeking and pleasure avoidance. What makes pleasure responsible is its impact on the other person or community, no doubt a judgement call. To the extent that the pleasure seeking enhances the other it is judged as responsible pleasure, to the extent that it causes harm to the other it is irresponsible pleasure. Indeed, Freud the hedonist believed that the pursuit of well-being was fundamentally the pursuit of individual sensual pleasure in a responsible context (Compton and Hoffman, 2020). As Compton and Hoffman (2020) note,

> A socially responsible form of hedonism, although regarding pleasure as the basic motivating force behind most human behavior, affirms that certain pleasures required positive social relationships with those close to us and with society at large.
>
> (p. 56)

For example, says Compton and Hoffman, some types of hedonism view family life or civic involvement as ways to maximize pleasure and contentment for all people involved. The goal here is to maximize the happiness for oneself and others. The good life in this version of hedonism is characterized in terms of positive emotions such as happiness, contentment, satisfaction, or joy (Compton and Hoffman, 2020).

In contrast, while the pursuit of pleasure may sometimes lead to an enhanced well-being, it is not always the case. For example, overindulgence in alcohol, drugs, and food may lead to addiction, cancer, and heart disease. Likewise, the pursuit of virtue may sometimes lead to pleasure, but on other occasions may not. For example, acts of courage, such as rescuing a person from drowning, or working hard to achieve success at a job that helps others may lead to pain rather than pleasure (Carr, 2022).

Perhaps the most important Freudian criticism of Koheleth's outlook on pleasure-seeking is the fact that Koheleth believes that because there is an endpoint to pleasure, namely, death, the accumulated pleasure is for naught. That is, pleasure is only regarded as ultimately satisfying if it, or its effects, lasts forever. This is an ill-conceived and ill-fated assumption that is common with those who have an episodically depressive or pessimistic outlook like Koheleth.

In his essay "On Transience" (1915/1916), in a dialogue with a poet (probably Rainer Maria Rilke),[2] Freud's main point is that the temporary nature of life and beauty, rather than reducing their value, in fact improves it by making us appreciate them more profoundly. Freud claims that the notion that the fleetingness of things should lead to despair (as with Koheleth) is a pessimistic assumption, and instead he suggests that it can actually motivate us to treasure the present moment. He uses a dialogue with the poet (who sounds similar to Koheleth, the poet), who expresses a more melancholic view on transience. Said Freud:

> I could not see my way to dispute the transience of all things, nor could I insist upon an exception in favour of what is beautiful and perfect. But I did dispute the pessimistic poet's view that the transience of what is beautiful involves any loss in its worth. On the contrary, an increase! Transience values is scarcity value in time. Limitation in the possibility of an enjoyment.
>
> (p. 305)

Freud believes that the knowledge of things being temporary can make us appreciate them more fully, like the beauty of a summer afternoon that will eventually fade with the approaching winter. Freud suggests that clinging to the past and lamenting loss is a form of mourning, and that we should be able to detach from lost objects to reinvest our libidinal energy in new ones. Incomplete mourning is when a person is unwilling and unable to move forward through the stages of grief (he is "stuck"), which can make it very hard to heal. As Rycroft (1995) notes, all schools of psychoanalysis believe that mourning is the normal analogue of depression, the loss in depression being not that of an actual person or thing, but an ambivalently invested "internal object" (a mental representation of a person or thing that has been internalized into a person's psyche, usually shaped in infancy and impacted on by parental caregivers). Said Freud:

> What spoilt their enjoyment of beauty must have been a revolt in their minds against mourning. The idea that all this beauty was transient was giving these sensitive minds a foretaste of mourning over its decrease; and, since the mind instinctively recoils from anything that is painful, they felt their enjoyment of beauty interfered with thoughts of its transience.
>
> (306)

Freud argues that a person's inability to truly appreciate beauty might emanate from an inordinate focus on the transience of things, delaying their ability to fully engage, mindfully, with the present moment and enjoy it. Koheleth appears to be in this category (although not in the carpe diem passages, of which there are seven! (Heim, personal communication)).

Responsible Pleasure

From a psychoanalytic point of view, the pursuit of sensible pleasure in everyday life is judged to be a "good" practice. All "schools" of psychoanalysis agree on this point. As I have said, Freud, for example, insisted "on the primacy of the drive theory [a view I am sympathetic to] and the version of the world associated with it, man as pleasure seeking" in an erotically tinged universe (Weinstein, 1990, p. 26). I have suggested, like in Freudian psychoanalysis, a degree of Epicurean hedonism and Stoic fatalism ("what will be, will be" while still taking responsible action within one's control) have their expression in Koheleth's philosophy of life. Putting aside his religious language and categories, his conclusion that the striving after pleasure and joy is a fundamental human motivation and goal is, of course, entirely compatible with the Freudian project. The questions that remain to be answered are what exactly constitutes meaningful and enduring pleasure and joy for Koheleth, how is it best attained, and what, beyond what we have already said, tends to work against experiencing it? It is impossible in this chapter to detail all of this, but a hint of what Koheleth has in mind may be helpful.

For Koheleth, like Freud, pleasure and joy are palpable, sensual, and concrete experiences. For example, Koheleth says, "Enjoy life with the woman whom you love." Koheleth is here advocating the importance of a love relationship (of any persuasion) and zestful and purposeful activity to attaining a degree of happiness. No psychoanalyst would disagree with this. However, what Koheleth adds here is rarely emphasized in the psychoanalytic narrative yet is an insight that can only heighten the satisfaction with love and purposeful activity. Following Freud, I am referring to the fact that the enjoyment of these experiences is enhanced by a greater mindfulness of the transitoriness of life. Moreover, it is this sense of resignation in the face of the brevity of life, in the face of life's all-too-frequent frustration and harshness, that makes these experiences that much more enjoyable and lasting. Such an attitude also fosters one of the most underrated sensibilities in the modern secular world, a sensibility that religious traditions have emphasized as fundamental to attaining a degree of happiness, a sense of gratitude for what one has. For Koheleth, a certain "downsizing" of one's infantile narcissism is a prerequisite for even episodic and praiseworthy pleasure, let alone a more solid and lasting sense of happiness and joy.

In contrast, Koheleth mocks the masses of people who choose to live their lives in a way that is not mindful of its tragic character as described throughout this book: the fragility and impermanence of human accomplishments; the uncertainty and lack of control of our destiny; the impossibility of achieving true knowledge, understanding, and insight into the world; and of course, the inevitability of death. These are the narcissists, and those for example who are driven by envy and greed, who do not embrace with melancholic resignation (though without despair) the absolute limitations on existence, and who have not cultivated a sense of gratitude for that which they have. Such people insist that they are masters of their own destiny, that through seeking and attaining more and more acquisitions they will forever be safe and happy.

In other words, in a number of different contexts, Koheleth criticizes the vanity of those who fetishize their existence. Fetishization, as I mean it, is "the organization of perception and action, by the personality, around a very striking and compelling – but narrow – theme," such as money (or as with Koheleth, other materialist pleasures) (Becker, 1969, p. 85). Such a person built him or herself firmly into his or her cultural world such that he or she is imprisoned in his or her own narrow behavioral mold. The reason a person artificially inflates a small area of the world and overvalues it, insinuates Koheleth, is that it represents an area that he or she can firmly hold on to, skillfully manipulate, and easily use to justify him or herself: his or her actions, sense of self, and options in the world. In psychoanalytic parlance, such a person is neurotic in that he or she demonstrates, for example, an extreme conceptual and behavioral poverty, blocking the forward momentum of action and the restriction of experience.

Koheleth is particularly hard on those who lust after wealth, the latter being common in our capitalist society. A "capitalist mind-set" is a mode of thinking that emphasizes individual self-interest, competition, and the quest for profit within a market economy:

> He who loves money will never have enough of it and he who loves wealth will never attain it – this is indeed vanity. For as wealth increases, so those

> who would spend it, hence what value is there in the owner's superior ability, except that he has more to look upon.
>
> (Gordis, 1951, p. 158, V. 9-VI. 9)

Koheleth is here critiquing those who make money, or symbolically any acquisition, the primary focus of self-value, the center of his or her universe.

Whether it is classical greed, diligence, or thrift (which for Koheleth is a sub-species of greed), or the quest after fame and power (which he says is frequently rooted in envy and the desire to compete and outdo others), Koheleth is making an insightful observation from which psychoanalysis could benefit: that the attempt to generate an absolute, closed, narrow, and concrete foundation to base and guide one's existence is ill-conceived, ill-advised, and ill-fated.

That is, in Koheleth's religious language, for example, through fetishization, the individual denies his or her creatureliness, denies God's transcendence and infinitude, and makes him or herself the Creator as he or she worships earthly things. Following Perry (1993), it is worth noting that for Koheleth, antithetical to contemporary viewpoints, it is the person of faith that is more open-minded and receptive than the man of experience. He is determinedly "unwilling to foreclose on God's nature or to infer the nature of things in general from particular human experience, no matter how broad and privileged." For such a person, the all of one's life, the totality of his acts, does not permit conclusions concerning the All (Perry, 1993, p. 35).

In the psychoanalytic lexicon, such a person is perhaps best described as a "malignant narcissist," as one who had developed a primary, self-centered, and driven hedonism that becomes an unhindered and toxic egoism. Malignant narcissism is a serious personality disorder that comprises a mixture of narcissism, antisocial behavior, and sadism. Individuals with malignant narcissism often express manipulative, aggressive, and abusive tendencies. Such a person forecloses any contact with a source of meaning which remains open, available, and untotalized, whether that meaning is called God or the Other (the latter may be a significant other, says Koheleth, "enjoy life with a woman you love"). In other words, the enjoyment and pleasure of, say, money, fame, power, and sex are ultimately empty and meaningless when they become fetishized, that is, become a neurotic fixation. However, following Levinas, enjoyment and pleasure can be more; they can be a basis for individuation when it is sanctioned by the consciousness of the other (Perry, 1993). And, says Levinas, to be conscious of the other mainly means to be responsible to and for the other. As Koheleth cautions us, "Remember your Creator in the days of your youth," that is, when pleasure and joy are most intense and motivating, as in youth, be mindful of the fact – and this is probably true even more so in the middle and especially old age – that it is the rooting of pleasure and joy in responsibility and care for the other that is likely to make them the most satisfying and meaningful. In other words, the striving after and attainment of money, fame, power, and sex are most likely to be sources of joy and not sources of the malevolent self-transformation, when they are knotted to the ethical relation. Moreover, it is the sense of gratitude, in religious language – a consciousness that God has provided us with the means of enjoyment – that encourages the prudent enjoyment of one's acquisitions and pleasures rather than degrading oneself or the other by the abuse of them (Cohen, 1970). As secular psychoanalyst Theodore Reik famously noted, "The sex urge hunts for lustful pleasure; while love is in search of joy and happiness."

Case Vignette

Galia, age 48, an Iranian Jewess, came to me once a week for about a year because she was depressed about the state of her life. "My life is out of control," "I have wasted my time for years," she told me. Galia said that she had wasted the last 20 years or so since she and her husband moved from Teheran to New York, with the expectation that they would move to Los Angeles once he finished his medical training in New York (about three years later). Galia had her family, her parents and two sisters, in Los Angeles, and she says that she missed them a lot. However, due to her husband's professional training, he secured a good job at one of the prestigious hospitals and has remained there ever since. Galia felt that her husband "owed" her due to her willingness to remain in New York for over 20 years rather than relocate to Los Angeles. While her husband was a very good provider, Galia felt there was something missing in the marriage for all those twenty years. She regarded her husband as a "good man," but not one that she felt passionately attracted to. While her obligations were to her husband, her romance lay elsewhere.

Galia was a high school teacher in Teheran, but once she came to New York she was a homemaker, having three children, two boys and one girl, who appeared to be flourishing in their lives, "thanks to my husband," Galia told me. He was a hands-on caregiver she said. Galia claimed that she was a lousy mother, not very nurturing nor stable. Her husband was very supportive of her, having encouraged her to recertify as a teacher, or do something else, that would make her happy, but she kept making excuses why she did "nothing" with her life for over two decades.

Galia described her upbringing in Teheran as a happy one. She claimed that her parents, her father was a real estate developer and her mother an accountant, were loving towards her and as having given her a good life. She said she was part of a tight-knit Jewish community in Teheran and did not feel any serious anti-Semitism while living in Iran. Her sisters were married with children and appeared to be flourishing in their lives.

While Galia said her marriage was not very good, her husband loved her, but she had an affair about a decade ago which almost busted up the marriage. Her husband hired a private investigator and had photographs to prove her infidelity. Despite the affair, her husband still loved Galia and wanted to give it another go.

Galia said that she stays in the marriage because her husband is a "good man," and he gives her a very materially comfortable life. They live in Manhattan in a three-bedroom apartment and are "well off."

Galia said the aforementioned affair was with an Iranian man who made it clear that their relationship was an affair, and there were no expectations of the relationship transitioning into something more serious (this man claimed he was happily married and had children). Once she and her husband were finished fighting about her affair (for many months), with him claiming that she did not love him anymore, Galia indicated to him that she would not be unfaithful again. She told her husband that she had the affair to experience increased excitement, something that her marriage of about 25 years lacked. While she dutifully slept with her husband, she said the sex was boring and usually fantasized about other men. Galia further indicated that all of her friends who had similar circumstances felt likewise.

What Galia did not tell her husband was that she was having numerous affairs with men for the last ten years, including multiple partners. Strangely, Galia had three men she was sleeping with each with the same name as her husband! Galia told me that the affairs satisfied her need for excitement and drama, and that she was unable to love, being self-centered and manipulative. "I don't know how to love," she told me, including her husband, even her children, whom she was dutiful but not particularly nurturing towards. "I probably should not have had kids," she told me. In fact, Galia indicated that the main appeal of her various affairs was to get the man to surrender to her charm and sexuality. Galia described herself as prone to jealousy when one of her lovers flirted with other women, or the man was attached to his mother, this motivating her to manipulate the man to want her. "I know how to control these men, to give me attention and affirmation. In truth I don't really care about any of them, it is like a big game to me."

In the transference, Galia treated me as a confidant, with no sign of her being seductive or controlling. I recently pointed out to her that while she had pleasure with the men she was sleeping with, getting orgasms, she still felt like there was something missing inside her. Galia responded by agreeing that the pleasure didn't last or make her feel good, telling me that she was "too broken to be fixed," that it is her nature to be unfaithful and have multiple partners. While Galia had pleasure with these other men, she in fact felt empty inside, leading to her seeking out one or other of her lovers for relief. And so, the pattern repeated itself. When I suggested to Galia that she come a second or even a third time each week, she was not interested, this probably being her way of controlling the proceedings and remaining at a safe distance. I felt that closeness and distance was one of Galia's core problems, and I had the distinct feeling that she kept me at an arm's distance.

The treatment is still ongoing, with Galia claiming that she knows there is something "seriously wrong" with her, but she "can't change." When I asked her why she felt so strongly that she could not change, at least in theory, she told me because "I don't really want to change, I know I will get caught again by my husband and that will be the end of the marriage." Galia appeared to believe her own words, though I thought that she often engaged in a delusional remolding of reality to suit her perverse desires.

So what manifestly looks like sexual pleasure is really a means of proving her power and control, none of it filling up the emptiness she feels inside, hence, doomed to repeat itself until the ultimate punishment of the marriage crashing and burning, that is, ending.

Notes

1 For many, the apparently unlimited hedonism is in tension with true wisdom; Heim believes that this is self-ironical (Heim, personal communication).
2 Razinsky (2015) notes that Freud was also walking with a third person, a speechless friend, who turned out to be the Russian-born psychoanalyst Lou Andreas Salome.

6 The Futility of Work

Said Koheleth early on in his book:

> I then turned to observe all the work that my hands had done, and all the labour I had strained to perform, and lo, everything was vanity and chasing of wind, with no advantage under the sun.
>
> (Gordis, 1951, p. 140, I. 2–11)

Koheleth was well aware that hard work makes up a sizeable part of one's everyday life. For most people, engaging in such work is not an option for one needs to make enough money to sustain oneself and one's family. Put simply, "we labor, toil and then die" (Gibson, 2017, p. 24).

As Gordis (1951) points out, Kohelet gives three reasons for people to work hard, all of them being susceptible to serious criticism. First is the joy of creation; it is rejected as a flimsy disguise for the competitive spirit by which man attempts to outdo his neighbor and rival. Said Koheleth:

> I saw that all hard work and skill are merely one's man's rivalry with his neighbor. This too is vanity and chasing the wind. Some men teach, "The fool folds his hands and thus destroys himself." But I declare: "Better a handful acquired with ease than two hands full gained through toil and chasing after wind."
>
> (Gordis, 1951, p. 150, IV. 4–16)

Fox (2004) aptly translates the Hebrew word for rivalry as envy. Envy in psychoanalytic parlance has been defined by Person et al. (2005) as the emotion connected with the notion that someone has something you very much want. Envy is, thus, a form of aggression since it expresses a wish not only to have what the other person has but to divest the person of what is treasured and make them suffer for having possessed it. Envy is often muddled with jealousy, which comprises three parties and has the aim of winning the exclusive love of the object over a rival for that love, and does not require the destruction of the rival.

DOI: 10.4324/9781003652816-6

For Koheleth the only reasonable course of action is to take one's ease in one's work. Workaholism, in other words, is ill-conceived and ill-advised. Rather, to engage in moderate work, perhaps with a sense of what we today call flow experience. Flow has been defined by the originator of the concept, Mihaly Csikszentmihalyi (1975):

> Flow denotes the holistic sensation present when we act with total involvement. . . . It is the state in which action follows upon action according to an internal logic which seems to need no conscious intervention on our part. We experience it as a unified flowing from one moment to the next, in which we feel in control of our actions, and in which there is little distinction between self and environment; between stimulus and response; or between past, present, and future.
>
> (p. 43)

Koheleth does not point to flow experience in his book, but the concept seems applicable to elaborating the notion of the ease of moderate work.

Second, Koheleth critically evaluates the alleged benefits of family companionship, which he regards as almost completely physical. That is, to literally provide one's family with their creature comforts. This rationale for hard work is found wanting. Said Koheleth:

> Men say, "Two are better than one, because they have a reward in their labour." True, for if either falls, the other can lift his comrade, but woe to him who is alone when he falls, with no one else to lift him. Then also, if two sleep together, they will be warm, but how can one alone keep warm? Moreover, if some enemy attack either one, the two will stand against him, while a triple cord cannot quickly be severed.
>
> (Gordis, 1951, p. 150, IV. 4–16)

As Fox (2004) points out, the word *labor* refers to life's activities and sufferings generally, and not simply to occupational labors or their earnings while engaging in their livelihood.

Thirdly is the claim that those who work hard to achieve fame are misguided for fame is a passing phenomenon. For example, a memorable deed or achievement is unknown in the ages before and after the achievement. A hundred years from now, most achievements are forgotten. Said Koheleth:

> "Better a lad of poor birth, who is wise, than an old king, who is a fool and can no longer take care of himself. For from the prison-house he came forth to rule, though he was born poor in the kingdom." I have seen all the living who walk under the sun on the side of the lad, his successor, who appears on the scene in his stead. Yet there is no end to the people who lived before

> them both, nor will later generations find joy in the youth – indeed, this, too, is vanity and chasing of wind.
>
> (Gordis, 1951, p. 152, IV. 4–16)

There are many psychological reasons why individuals seek out fame. For example, to achieve an upsurge of self-esteem (i.e., a narcissistic motivation), often emanating from a desire for attention, validation, a sense of importance, social influence, and sometimes even a need to surmount feelings of insecurity or neglect (i.e., a poor self-concept), with the appeal of allure and privilege acting as other motivations, particularly in today's social media–driven world where fame appears to be more reachable than ever before.

Finally, Koheleth seems to be describing, or at least pointing to, those individuals who suffer from "burnout." Burnout emanates from inordinate demands with inadequate support and supervision (Carr, 2022). Burnout is characterized by emotional, mental, and physical exhaustion due to stress associated with the specific work one is doing. Koheleth appears to be unable (and/or unwilling) to conceptualize those individuals who relate to their work as a "calling," a source of personal fulfillment and meaning, including them believing that what they did had a socially useful function (Carr, 2022). I am reminded of a patient of mine who helped build/repair bridges in New York City. He told me that he loved his work and felt proud that he was contributing to the safety and well-being of his fellow New Yorkers.

There are other important aspects of the psychology of work that Koheleth does not mention let alone reflect upon. It is here that psychoanalysis has its main contribution.

Psychoanalysis and Work

Freud, too, reflected on the meaning of work:

> I could not contemplate with any sort of comfort a life without work. Creative imagination and work go together with me; I take no delight in anything else.
>
> (Freud, 1910/1963, p. 35)

And Freud also noted:

> But she [Nature] endowed me with a dauntless love of truth, the keen eye of an investigator, a rightful sense of the values of life, and the gift of working hard and finding pleasure in doing so.
>
> (Jones, 1953–1957, p. 118)

And finally:

> A man like me cannot live without a hobby-horse, without a consuming passion, without – in Schiller's words – a tyrant. I have found one ["working well, writing well"]. In its service I know no limits.
>
> (1985/1995, p. 129)

Freud, Erik Erikson tells us, said that "to love and work" were the central therapeutic goals of psychoanalysis, these being the twin pillars of a sound mind and for living the "good life" (Erikson, 1959, p. 96).[1] Indeed, psychoanalysis is full of work metaphors, many first used by Freud, such as "analytic work, dream work, mourning work, joke work, working through" (and Ralph Greenson's notion of "working alliance"), reinforcing the notion that "adult maturity" involves a robust capacity to work effectively (Blum, 1997, p. 19).[2] Freud's views of work, however, were hardly clear and consistent, though his ambiguous and ambivalent formulations were the precursors to most psychoanalytic theorizing on work behavior.

As Neff notes (1965, p. 325), on the one hand, Freud claims that along with love, work is the great realm of human activity that helps us comprehend the nature of human society:

> The communal life of human beings had . . . a twofold foundation: the compulsion to work, which was created by external necessity, and the power of love. . . . Eros and Ananke [Love and Necessity] have become the parents of human civilization.
>
> (Freud, 1930/1961, p. 101)

In Freud's view, work allowed humans to be "able to live together in a community" with a minimum of discord and hostility (Freud, 1930/1961, p. 101). Moreover, he said, there is an economic motivator for human society in that humanity "does not possess enough provisions to keep its members alive unless they work," so "it must restrict the number of its members and divert their energies from sexual activity to work" (Freud, 1916–1917, p. 312). On the other hand, Freud did not view work as inherently pleasurable activity in which man wanted to engage, but rather a hardship, a burdensome, if not painful, obligation to be endured (Neff, 1965, p. 325). Said Freud, "Men are not spontaneously fond of work" and therefore require a certain amount of societal "coercion and renunciation of instinct" (1927, p. 8). Indeed, Mark Twain affirmed Freud's observation when he famously quipped, "Work is a necessary evil to be avoided" (www.quoteworld.org › Mark Twain, retrieved

3/1/25). Freud explains why work is so objectionable in terms of his understanding of the human condition:

> Human beings exhibit an inborn tendency to carelessness, irregularity and unreliability in their work . . . a laborious training is needed before they learn to follow the example of their celestial models.
>
> (Freud, 1930/1961, p. 93)

What Freud is getting at here is now common knowledge – growing up requires relinquishing the childhood caste of mind, one that is geared toward maximizing pleasure and avoiding unpleasure, the "pleasure principle," in favor of living according to the "reality principle." The reality principle requires that one no longer live according to the demands of immediate gratification of one's needs and wishes, but rather a reasonable and self-preserving evaluation of the external world governs decision-making in the service of pleasure-attainment. Indeed, Freud was well aware that perhaps more than anything else humans do, it is work that lodges a human being in the totality of "real" things in the world – in "actual" being and existence: "No other technique for the conduct of life attaches the individual so firmly to reality as laying emphasis on work; for his work at least gives him a secure place in a portion of reality, in the human community" (Freud, 1930/1961, p. 80).

Moreover, Freud continues, work can be gratifying, at least in terms of "the economics of the libido":

> The possibility that work offers of displacing a large amount of libidinal components, whether narcissistic, aggressive or even erotic, on to professional work and on to the human relations connected with it lends it a value by no means second to what it enjoys as something indispensable to the preservation and justification of existence in society. Professional activity is a source of special satisfaction if it is a freely chosen one if . . . by means of sublimation, it makes possible the use of existing inclinations, of persisting or constitutionally reinforced instinctual impulses.
>
> (Freud, 1930/1961, p. 80)

While Freud acknowledges previously that work can provide a modicum of personal satisfaction (e.g., a sense of competence and mastery), he nevertheless concludes that for most people, it is hardly the "royal road" to the "good life":

> And yet, as a path to happiness, work is not highly prized by men. They do not strive after it as they do after other possibilities of satisfaction. The great majority of people only work under the stress of necessity, and this natural human aversion to work raises most difficult social problems.
>
> (Freud, 1930/1961, p. 80)

What Freud is claiming regarding the function of work is in sync with his general view of the human condition – namely, that there is a painful dialectic between culture and desire, one in which most of the time the individual has to repudiate his instinctual life, his sexual and aggressive wishes, and adapt to living according to the reality principle, both for the sake of individual and collective survival. Perhaps this is most evident in terms of the parent/child relationship in which parents try to civilize their children, that is, tame their sexual and aggressive tendencies through a range of child-rearing strategies and tactics, including those that take advantage of the child's vulnerability, his need for love and support and his fear of losing it.

For Freud, then, broadly speaking, individuals work because they have to survive, and this self-preservation requires effectively managing those pressing demands emanating from external circumstances (e.g., society's rules and norms of permissible conduct) and internal sources (e.g., sexual and aggressive wishes). The great English playwright Noel Coward captured the main thrust of Freud's view in terms of everyday life: "Your motivation is your pay packet on Friday. Now get on with it" (Fadiman and Brand, 1985, p. 146).

Drawing from the vocational and organizational psychology literatures, a very useful way of applying Freud's advice is to conceive of choosing a career – listen to "the deep inner needs of our nature," the unconscious (Reik, 1983, p. 7) – is in terms of a "calling," as opposed to a "job" or "career." As sociologists Bellah and colleagues (1986) first pointed out in their bestselling book, *Habits of the Heart: Individualism and Commitment in American Life,*[3] a person with a "job" orientation to work is geared toward earning a living for him and his family to prosper and to maximize their amount of leisure time. In other words, work is viewed strictly as a practical means to a financial end. Moreover, his sense of self is mainly defined by financial success, security, "and all that money can buy" (p. 66). A "career" is a way to advance oneself in terms of accomplishment, status, and prestige. Such people mainly work in order to move up the hierarchical ladder, to be promoted, a competitive process they very much enjoy. The sense of self that is associated with a career is characterized by a broader kind of success than a job in that by attaining a degree of expanding power and competency, work itself becomes a way of sustaining self-esteem (Bellah et al., 1986). Individuals who have a "job" and "career" orientation toward work tend to have personal identities that do not significantly overlap with the actual work they do; to a large extent they view what they do at work as distinct from the rest of their life (Berg et al., 2010, p. 974). They narrate their lives in terms of having a "work self" and a "non-work self," and rarely do they feel they are a "whole" or "complete self."

In contrast, a "calling" is a work orientation in which a person views their work as deeply satisfying and socially beneficial. That is, an individual chooses an occupation that he "feels drawn to pursue," often powerfully. He anticipates it to be "intrinsically enjoyable and meaningful," especially as a socially useful endeavor, and he views it "as a central part of his identity"

(Berg et al., 2010, p. 973). As Bellah and colleagues noted, such work "constitutes a practical ideal of activity and character that makes a person's work morally inseparable from his or her life," and it links the person not only more intensely to his co-workers but to the larger community (Berg et al., 2010, p. 973).

Freud further elaborated the benefits of work:

> [N]o other technique for the conduct of life attaches the individual so firmly to reality as laying emphasis on work; for his work at least gives him a secure place in a portion of reality, in the human community.
>
> (1930/1961, p. 80)

What Freud is getting at appears to be straightforward. Psychoanalytically work has some of the following benefits to the individual. As Akhtar points out, work is not the same thing as maintaining a job, or earning money, though it may include them; it requires physical or mental activity designed to bring about a preferred outcome; it tends to bring about "narcissistic, object related, sexualized, and aggressive pleasure but these are secondary, since work has its own rewards for the ego," such as work being pleasurable for its own sake and a context for forgetting oneself (Phillips, 2021); work helps regulate self-esteem and contributes to identity maintenance; "it follows a developmental line from infancy to old age with the phases of latency and young adulthood being the most important to its consolidation" (Akhtar, 2009, p. 308).

Case Vignette

Richard, age 70, came to me because he was depressed about his life. His marriage was lousy, he and his wife lived like two ships passing in the night. He couldn't remember the last time he had sexual relations with his estranged wife. He also had numerous affairs that were ultimately unsatisfying he told me. Richard came from a nuclear family in which his mother was passive but dutiful and a father who was a successful financial consultant. He described his father in rather cold terms, telling me that while his father made a lot of money, he was not particularly supportive of his son's aspirations to be in the family business. Instead, his father was engaged in government, once briefly running for office, which he lost. Richard had two children, a daughter who became a family lawyer and a son who was something of a "rolling stone," who Richard had hoped would have taken over his very successful financial consultancy (at least successful by conventional standards). Richard had a lousy relationship with his daughter and a "cool" relationship with his wayward son.

Richard was a multimillionaire, though as he told me, he felt he was "a failure," not being wealthy like his father who died prematurely of a brain aneurism when Richard was about age 40. Richard had one brother whom he was estranged from, and he did not have any close friends, pushing people away who wanted to be his friend. Richard described himself "as lonely for years."

From what I could discern, Richard had a bad case of anhedonia, the inability to experience pleasure in normal activities that most people felt good about. Instead the only thing that made him feel vital and temporarily satisfied was making "big deals" in his merger and acquisition business. In fact, Richard told me that he was "like a drug addict," that is, he only "got turned on" by making the successful "big deals." While Richard was a multimillionaire he felt that he "never made it really big" like some of his colleagues. He also said that compared to his father, he wasn't very successful. I commented on the unresolved Oedipal issues, though it did not change him much.

In the twice-a-week treatment that went on for about a year (Richard bolted without saying good-bye as it were, and he never paid his last bill), Richard repeatedly complained that he never made it "in the big leagues." That is, Richard compared himself with the near billionaires whom he knew in the same business, feeling that he was "in the little league." In fact, just about all that Richard could talk about was his "lack of success" and blaming his father for not helping him, including taking over his father's business, which would have put him in the "big league." It seemed as if part of his inability to be content and grateful for how well he had done financially was that it allowed him to keep being angry with his father. A feeling he hung on to tenaciously.

Richard viewed me in the transference with a degree of suspicion, feeling that I was not very useful as a therapist since I could not make him feel financially successful, nor shift his obsessive focus on making a lot of money as a basis of his self-value. In fact, the only thing that excited him was making the deal and earning a lot of money, which had become fetishized. That is, having an extreme and irrational commitment to, or obsession with money. Richard repeatedly complained that he was not as rich as the "big gorillas," and he admitted that competing with his colleagues and striving for ever more and more financial success was the only thing that ultimately mattered to him. "It turns me on," said Richard.

Richard was rather obsessed with the fact that his father, an extremely rich man, never lifted a finger to help him in his own merger and acquisitions business. When I pointed out that Richard felt competitive with his father, he clarified that he was not competitive with him as much as angry at his father for not doing the right thing and letting him into the family business. In fact, Richard tearfully told me that his father more or less "cut" him out of his will, leaving him with a small amount of money. Richard's mother, passive in the extreme, was under the control of her husband and often did his bidding.

For the most part, the only thing that validated Richard was the love of money, as earned by making the "big deal." In fact, I never was able to get him off the single track he was on: Richard fantasized earning millions of dollars after closing the deal, this being the only thing that validated him. Indeed,

Richard complained that business had greatly slowed down, and as a result he "didn't know what to do with" himself. He spent most of his time looking for the next deal, having given up on his wife and children as meaning-giving, affect-integrating, and action-guiding entities.

From what I could determine, Richard was a "soldier in search of a war," that is, he was very angry at his father, feeling that he never helped reach the apex of financial success. While making money and closing the big deal was the only thing that mattered to him, Richard acknowledged that his depressed feeling was irrational, that he had enough money to retire and live happily ever after, he nevertheless harped on the fact that he was essentially "a loser." Richard was thus in a state of incomplete mourning. Not only for his place in the big leagues and the fantasy of his son taking over the business, but for never having fully grieved the loss of his father, whom he was still very angry with for not supporting him in the family business, nor teaching him about it. In this context, work was the only activity that this very sad man had that potentially made him feel a modicum of fleeting happiness. Richard, then, was a tragic character, who had everything, as it were, but felt like he had nothing.

Notes

1 Gedo believed that Freud was "excessively careerist" in his viewpoint. Gedo claims that Freud would have been less tied to his bourgeois socio-economic values and more psychologically right if he simply put forth the notion that mental health required the "freedom from any incapacity" to love and work. Indeed, there are normative circumstances where it is not unhealthy to work, such as in retirement (1997, pp. 134, 133).

2 As Freud noted in his *Introductory Lectures on Psychoanalysis*, "The distinction between nervous health and neurosis is thus reduced to a practical question and is decided by the outcome – by whether the subject is left with a sufficient amount of capacity for enjoyment and efficiency" (1916–1917, p. 457).

3 Amy Wrzesniewski et al. (1997) have researched this tripartate way of conceptualizing work and have confirmed Bellah et al.'s (1986) findings.

7 The Futility of Love

Koheleth did not have much to say about the love relationship, though he seemed to have believed that a man should have a female partner, one that provided nurturance and stability (note the heterosexual bias). As Fox (2004) observed, "In spite of his acrid comments about women in 7:24–29, Koheleth does not think it is a good for a man to be alone. A man should share his life with a female companion" (p. 63). This being said, there is no evidence that Koheleth was married, and chances are that he had a number of relationships that were not successful, ultimately ending up alone and disenchanted or worse. Gordis (1951) suggests, or rather speculates, that Koheleth did not trust women, possibly because of his disappointing relationships. Fox (2004) also claims that Koheleth's negativity towards women was in part due to him not having any successful love relationship.

Koheleth had a duality of structure when it comes to the problem of love. First, he says the following:

> I find woman more bitter than death, for her heart is full of traps and snares, her hands are chains. He who is favoured by God will escape her, but the sinner will be trapped by her.
>
> See, this I have found, says Koheleth, as I sought, step by step, to reach a conclusion. This, too, I sought but in vain, one[upright] man in a thousand I did find, but one woman among as many I could not find. Besides, note this that I have learnt: God has made men straightforward, but they have sought out many devices.
>
> (Gordis, 1951, p. 170, VII. 26–29)

As this passage indicates, Koheleth had a fairly grim view of men, "one [upright] man in a thousand I did find." However, he seems to have thought even worse of women, not really having faith in them, "not . . . one [upright] woman among as many I could not find" (Gordis, 1951).

DOI: 10.4324/9781003652816-7

In contrast, and towards the end of the book, Koheleth says the following:

Go, then, eat your bread with joy,
And drink your wine with a glad heart,
For God has already approved your actions.
At all times let your clothes be white, [a festive clothing signifying purity and innocence]
And oil on your head not be lacking.

Enjoy the life with the woman whom you love,
Through all the vain days of your life,
Which God has given you under the sun,
Throughout your brief days,
For that is your reward in life
For your toil under the sun
(Gordis, 1951, p. 178, IX. 4–12)

In the aforementioned first passage Koheleth appears to be describing woman as the consummate femme fatale. That is, an attractive and seductive woman, particularly one who is likely to cause emotional suffering or disaster to a man who becomes involved with her. Based on this passage, Koheleth has been described as misogynistic by some scholars (Seow, 1997). Indeed, Koheleth is here expressing a view of woman that regards her as controlling if not castrating, perhaps motivated by malevolence and the like. Fox (2004) believes this passage "is clearly hyperbolic" (p. 51).

The second aforementioned quotation describes woman in a somewhat idealized manner, as providing him with personal satisfaction. Joining the passages, it calls to mind a man who may be suffering from the Madonna-whore complex. As Freud, the originator of the concept, famously said, "Where they love they do not desire and where they desire they cannot love" (1912, p. 183). In the Madonna-whore complex some heterosexual men can only view women as one or the other, and never integrate these two perceptions into the same person. So in his unconscious mind, such men either view a woman as pure and good, as a saint-like mother, or as debased whores. Men with this complex desire a sexual partner who has been degraded (whore) while they cannot desire the respected partner (Madonna). The reasons for this, according to Freud, is that there is a division between the affectionate and the sexual tendencies in male desire. Oedipal and castration anxiety fears prohibit the affection felt for previous incestuous objects (the mother) from being attached to women who are sensually desired (the whore). Indeed, Freud, too, found love relationships very challenging.

He once said to the French author and psychoanalyst Princess Maria Bonaparte, "The great question that has never been answered, and which I have not yet been able to answer, despite my thirty years of research into the feminine soul, is 'What does a woman want?'" (Jones, 1953, vol. 2, p 421).

"Enjoy the life with the woman whom you love," says Koheleth. Presumably, at the time this was written, this meant being married to a woman whom one felt deep and abiding affection, and who got along in terms of everyday life. Koheleth does not detail what he meant by the aforementioned, that is, what constitutes such love. Perhaps because he probably did not easily trust women, he kept his observations to a minimum. It is the flip side of his ambivalence towards women putting aside all of his negativity towards women. What is unclear is how he transitions from one view to the other.

What is clear, however, is that Koheleth's notion of a love relationship had "the self . . . to be the measure of all things" (Crenshaw, 1987, p. 82). That is, the aim of love was to satisfy the self in terms of sexual desire and comfort. There are, however, different ways of conceptualizing love relationships in contrast to Koheleth's aim of self-gratification; for example, following Levinas, what is important is to assume that one is an ethical subject. The ethical subject is not a rational, self-contained being, but is one who is fundamentally oriented towards and responsible for the other, a responsibility that emanates from a pre-ontological, pre-rational encounter with the "Face of the Other" (the irreducible otherness of the other, a presence that demands acknowledgement and responsibility).

Says Levinas, the love commandment (love your neighbor as yourself), which Koheleth probably believed in, "still assumes the prototype of love to be love of oneself," that is, "self-love is accepted as the very definition of a person." Rather, Levinas's ethic asserts, "Be responsible for the other as you are responsible for yourself" (Levinas, 1987, p. 225). Levinas thus invites us to consider the cultivation of "goodness" as a guiding metaphor. "Goodness," he says "consists in taking up a position such that the Other counts more than myself" (1969, p. 247). Such a position of being-for-the-other is foreign to Koheleth's worldview.

What gets in the way of having a flourishing love relationship? For Koheleth, it was in part his general view of them. He claims women are "more bitter than death," they are "full of traps and snares," and their "hands are chains." The aforementioned is a very cynical and dark view of women. With such a perception of the nature of women, it is nearly impossible to have a plausible love relationship. Fortunately for Koheleth, this is only one side of his ambivalent attitude towards women.

For Koheleth, what thwarts love relationships is the chasing after transitory earthly pleasures and the intrinsic futility of life, leading to an emphasis on personal gain (e.g., wealth, fame) and ignoring the importance of cherishing authentic connection and empathic companionship. It is noteworthy that nearly 50% of marriages will end in divorce or separation. Marriages can fail due to a mixture of limitations, including lack of commitment, unfaithfulness, communication difficulties, frequent bickering, financial conflicts, and a waning in intimacy.

Koheleth stresses the vanity of worldly pursuits, suggesting that material possessions and accomplishments ultimately offer little enduring satisfaction. This can lead individuals to prioritize these things over authentic relationships, which are regarded as more precious and enduring.

Koheleth suggests that there is an inclination for people to become extremely self-regarding, focusing on satisfying their own narcissistic desires and ambitions rather than the needs and well-being of others. This self-centric outlook can create obstacles to creating/finding healthy and satisfying relationships. Such an inclination is in sync with Freud's outlook on the human condition. As Freud wrote to American neurologist James Jackson Putnam on 6/17/1915:

> The unworthiness of human beings, including the analyst, always impressed me deeply, but why should analyzed men and women in fact be better. Analysis makes for integration but does not itself make for goodness.
>
> (Hale, 1971, p. 188)

And again, in an 8/7/1915 letter to Putnam:

> When I ask myself why I have always striven honestly to be considerate of other and if possible kind to them and why I did not give this up when I noticed that one is harmed by such behavior and is victimized because others are brutal and unreliable, I really have no answer. It surely was not the sensible thing to do.
>
> (Hale, 1971, pp. 189–190)

And finally, in a letter to Swiss pastor Oscar Pfister:

> I don't cudgel my brains much about good and evil, but I have not found much good in the average human being. Most of them are in my experience riff-raff, whether they loudly proclaim this or that ethical doctrine or none at all.
>
> (Jones, 1953/1957, vol. 2, p. 457)

These quotations depict Freud's pessimism at its most extreme, believing as did Koheleth that most people are profoundly compromised beings.

Ecclesiastes 4:9–12 stresses the advantages of having a life-partner, emphasizing the joint support and strength that emanate from working together and facing challenges and difficulties as a unit ("two are better than one," "if either falls, the other can lift his comrade," "if two sleep together, they will be warm"). This suggests that not nurturing such relationships and choosing to be on one's own can lead to a less satisfying and purposeful life. In the USA, a significant amount of the adult population chooses to remain single, with nearly 40% of adults living without a spouse or partner, a number that has increased from 29% in 1990.

As I have indicated in Chapter 6 on the futility of work, Ecclesiastes 4:4–16 cautions against forgoing personal relationships on the altar of work and wealth, stressing that people and human connections are more significant than material acquisitions or accomplishments. Koheleth also advocates mindfulness, finding joy in the present moment and enjoying life's simple pleasures, including human relationships, rather than continually questing for more. Thus, Koheleth believed that a wholesome balance between work, accomplishment, and relationships, is essential for a satisfying or flourishing life.

A strong relationship is built on, for example, trust, safety, and faith, where each partner is honest and dedicated to the best interests of the other. Ecclesiastes 4:9–12 suggests that marriage is a partnership based on mutual support and strength, where two people can lift each other up and endure hardships together. Studies have found that married people in general report higher levels of happiness and well-being compared to their unmarried counterparts, with marriage being a strong predictor of happiness.

For Koheleth, a strong union needs to be based on a commitment to God, where both partners are able to rejoice in the good times and endure the bad times together. Some interpretations of Ecclesiastes suggest that a strong relationship, including marriage, is a partnership based on, for example, the aforementioned trust, safety, and faith, with God as a third element that strengthens the connection. As Levinas says, "Through my relation to the Other, I am in touch with God" (1989, p. 17). And Buber observes, the I-Thou relationship with God, the Eternal Thou, serves as a model for and potentiates authentic relationships between human beings.

I want to remind the reader that the last six verses of the book of Ecclesiastes was, most scholars believe, written by an orthodox editor who probably was a friend or colleague of Koheleth but was distressed by his skepticism. While these verses were an attempt at damage-control, I think the editor unconsciously actually wrote verses that capture the very core of what Koheleth believed and advocated, and they should be regarded as integral and consistent with the rest of the book, at least my reading of the book of Ecclesiastes:

> In sum, having heard everything, fear God and keep His commandments, for that is man's whole duty. For God will bring every deed to judgment, upon everything hidden whether it be good or evil.
>
> (Gordis, 1951, p. 190, XII. 9–14)

Despite all the uncertainty, ignorance, conflicts, and angst, Koheleth believed that practice should not wait for theory just as life so often does not wait for understanding and insight (Guthrie and Motyer, 1970, p. 578). What really matters and determines whether one's relationship is futile or meaningful, what perhaps makes life the most meaningful, is the ethical relation, which means as Koheleth has taught us, creating joy that is rooted and expressed in responsibility to, and for, the other.

Psychoanalytic Musings on Love

There is a crucial problem in the psychoanalytic and other scholarly literature on love. That is, what is love anyway? I have no intention of entering deeply into the problems of the definitions and meanings of love for it would require many volumes even to scrape the surface. However, it is important that the reader understand that there is no consensus with regards to defining and understanding the term and the experience(s) it allegedly refers to. Thus, the straightforward, though clearly limited, *The Concise Oxford Dictionary*'s definition of love is probably the best place to begin our discussion: "an intense feeling of deep affection or fondness for a person or thing; great liking" (Allen, 1990, p. 708).

To make matters even more complicated, there are many forms of love, each with its own phenomenology and psychodynamics. For example, there is love of wife/ husband/significant other, child, parent, God, knowledge, beauty, country, a cause, humanity, brotherly love, and according to Freud, possibly the purest of all love relations love for our pet! Says Freud,

> It really explains why we can love an animal . . . with such extraordinary intensity; affection without ambivalence, the simplicity of a life free from the almost unbearable conflict of civilization, the beauty of an existence complete in itself . . . Often when stroking Jo-fi [his dog] I have caught myself humming a melody which, unmusical as I am, I can't help recognizing as the aria from *Don Giovanni*: "a bond of friendship unites us both."
> (Steadman, 1979, p. 108)[1]

Whether Freud meant exactly what he said is not clear, but he was pointing to strong friendship as one of the clearest expressions of a "higher level" form of love, of what Aristotle called "perfected" love. Aristotle indicated that friendships (i.e., love) are shaped and sustained on different bases. There are those who sustain friendship mainly for the sensual gratification it provides; others sustain friendship for reasons of usefulness, and finally, there are friendships that are lodged in virtue. That is, one wants for one's friend what is most beneficial for one's friend. Such friendship is "perfected," says Aristotle, *telia philia*, in that its goals and aspirations, its objective, does not go beyond the friendship itself. It facilitates the good. Needless to say, such friendships are neither easily created nor common.[2] Roughly speaking, the Freudian construal of love most resonates with the first two forms of Aristotle's friendship, though obviously the matter is hardly so clear or simple. Our focus in this section will be on the ideal form of love between two adults, at least as psychoanalytic perspectives tend to construe it, that is, what analysts sometimes call "healthy," "mature," or "authentic" "object love." Briefly, object love depicts the self's cluster of emotions and attitudes towards "integrated whole objects" (e.g., significant others) that is the basis, the source of its gratification and pleasure (Moore and Fine, 1990, p. 129).

For Freud, as for all subsequent psychoanalysts, love has been approached mainly from the point of view of describing and understanding that which interferes and corrupts the capacity to love. And this is one of the connections to Koheleth, who also was concerned with what subverts love. Indeed, there is no body of knowledge that better depicts what St. Augustine called "disordered love," a lack of psychological fit between various human needs and wishes and the objects that can gratify them (Marcus, 2003). While psychoanalysis has in general been unsurpassable in explicating that which undermines mature love, it has been much weaker in depicting what constitutes and sustains it. What follows are some of the most interesting contributions of psychoanalysis to understanding what constitutes healthy/mature love relations (and secondarily, what corrupts it).

For Freud, all love relations are a "refinding of the object," roughly analogous to the emotional experience of symbiotic togetherness with the mother or caregiver (Moore and Fine, 1990, p. 113). What this means in terms of establishing love relations is that to some extent the choice of our significant other repeats or calls to mind aspects of our childhood caregivers. Love, says Freud, "consists of new editions of old traits and it repeats infantile reactions" (Freud, 1914/1915, p. 168). That is, all love is based on infantile templates, fundamentally a fixation on the parents, what Freud calls transference love. According to Reuben Fine, transference love and ordinary love only differ in terms of degree (Fine, 1979, p. 48). The problem with this is that if we refind that which is "bad" from our childhood experiences, it usually leads to impoverished and/or destructive intimate relationships. The trick, then, is to refind in the significant other that which is consciously and unconsciously "good" from our childhood caregivers, so that my partner and I have a better chance of being happy in our love relation.

For Freud, however, to accomplish this seemingly straightforward task is not at all simple for it requires resolving at a higher level of personality integration at least three aspects of love: "narcissistic versus object love, infantile versus mature love, and love versus hate" (Moore and Fine, 1990, p. 113). To the extent that love is dominated by inordinate, unhealthy, and pathological narcissism (e.g., self-centeredness and selfishness), infantile and dependent wishes and behavior (e.g., the other exists mainly to gratify one's needs and wishes on demand) and hate (e.g., heightened ambivalence), one's love relation is doomed to failure. To the extent that it is animated by altruistic concerns (e.g., enhancing the other), is mature (e.g., the recognition that the separate other has needs and wishes worthy of gratifying), and is mainly affectionate (e.g., not corrupted by aggression), it is likely to succeed (Moore and Fine, 1990). For Freud, and this needs to be emphasized, all relationships are ambivalent, at least to some extent. In this sense Koheleth's ambivalence about women is in sync with Freud's formulation. However, ultimately, the precondition to maintain a stable, healthy, mature love relation is that affectionate sentiments towards one's significant other are, in general, much stronger and pervasive than the aggressive ones. Towards the end of the book of Ecclesiastes, Koheleth appears to be less ambivalent about women and their capacity to make him happy ("Enjoy the life with the woman whom you love").

For Freud, love is understood within his closed energy-driven model and instinct-dominated outlook. All forms of love are seen as derivatives of instinct, and their function is to give instinctual gratification. In a sense then, for Freud all love is love of a need-satisfying object. Mature object love, in contrast to infantile, dependent, need-satisfying love, is love that recognizes the reality of the other, his otherness, that he is a separate person with needs and wishes requiring and deserving gratification. Perhaps most importantly, for Freud the capacity for mature love requires object constancy, the capability to maintain an enduring relationship with a specific, single, separate other. This in turn presupposes the development of both a stable, structurally sound, coherent self and secure internalized object relations. Normal love, says Freud, thus results from the blending of caring, affectionate and sexual feelings toward a person of the opposite sex. Its accomplishment is characterized by genital primacy in sexuality and by object love in relationships with others (Freud, 1905).[3]

For Freud, love relations, actually all human relations, largely reflect a utilitarian motive, that of using the other to gratify biologically endowed drives as means to one's end. Ginsberg notes, Koheleth "recommends generosity with a purely utilitarian motivation (one will then be more likely to be shown generosity if one should ever need it)" (Ginsberg, 1969, p. 55). As Kleinian analyst Donald Meltzer points out, for Freud, love is like opening up a factory, of making a kind of capital investment bent on generating a profit. One does not invest one's libido unless one feels fairly sure that one will get back more than one gives (Alford, 1998, p. 128). For Klein, on the other hand, love is conceptualized more in terms of bequeathing a charity (Alford, 1998, p. 128). That is, says Alford, "love gets from the very act of giving. It gets the opportunity to repair the self by repairing and restoring the world, or at least a little part of it" (Alford, 1998, p. 128). For Klein, love emanates from the infant's sense of gratitude toward the "good" mother, in Kleinian language, toward the satisfying, "good breast." This feeling is the basis for the infant's and later the adult's "appreciation of all goodness in the self and in others" (Bergmann, 1987, p. 248). By the end of the book of Ecclesiastes he appears to embrace a *carpe diem* outlook, which is another way of speaking about embracing life without reserve.

For Freud, love was perhaps the most important way of obtaining happiness, giving and receiving love; the "union of mental and bodily satisfaction in the enjoyment of love is one of its [life's] culminating peaks" (Freud, 1914/1915, p. 169). Koheleth would agree with this. Love is also, says Freud, crucial because it underpins other extremely important aspects of life and civilization. For instance, it libidinally binds and animates ones ties to family, friends, community, and to the world at large. Without the force of Eros, Freud's poetic metaphor for the life-force and sexual instincts, civilization is doomed to be overwhelmed by the inherent aggressiveness and destructiveness that constitutes Thanatos, the Death Instinct.

Psychoanalysis has of course developed its theories of love since Freud in interesting ways, and I want to briefly touch upon some of these contributions. This mini-survey is meant to be illustrative not comprehensive.

Erik H. Erikson, the great ego psychologist, describes love as the key virtue, as the ego strength that emerges after successful resolution of the intimacy versus isolation ego crisis, the sixth stage of human development of the life cycle. Erikson defines love as "mutuality of devotion forever subduing the antagonisms inherent in divided function" (Erikson, 1964, p. 129). Love thus involves a complementarity of identities, having both the ego strength to share identity for "mutual verification" of selected identity, and drawing from the supportive and nurturing other "the strength to be 'self-ish'" (Monte, 1980, p. 256).

Heinz Kohut's psychoanalytic self-psychology claims that love is fundamentally establishing a "selfobject." A selfobject is someone who strengthens and sustains the sense of self, the self's cohesion, firmness, and harmony (Kohut, 1984, p. 49). In infantile love the significant other, the selfobject, mainly functions for my benefit and survival, a template rooted in early childhood experience of the empathic, supportive, reassuring, and approving "good" mother or caregiver. In mature love the self is better grounded, sustained, and strengthened and thus capable of a more intense experience of receiving and giving love. In other words, for Kohut, in the love relationship one refinds the good mother, the selfobject, the one who calls to mind, sustains, and strengthens structural self-coherence, energic vigor, aliveness, and integration and balance among the diverse elements of the self. For the love relationship to work, both people need to refind the self-selfobject relationships they had in their parent/caregiver-to-child relationships. For Kohut, the sense of comfort, healing, and happiness that characterizes the best of love is precisely the byproduct of this mutual self-selfobject refinding. Koheleth seems to think likewise.

Finally, Jacques Lacan says it is "impossible to say anything meaningful" or intelligible about love (Evans, 1996, p. 103).[4] This calls to mind the dark side of Koheleth's attitude towards women. For Lacan, love must be understood in terms of what he views as the larger ethical goal of psychoanalysis, namely, the discovery of the reality and truth of the Unconscious and its powerful interpretive grip over the subject (Fryer, 2004, p. 190). Thus, as Evans points out, Lacan says love is situated as a "purely imaginary phenomenon" although it has an impact in the symbolic register (Evans, 1996, p. 103).[5] Love for Lacan "is autoerotic" and mainly has a "narcissistic structure" since "its one's own ego that one loves in love, one's own ego made real on the imaginary level" (Bowie, 1991, p. 103).[6] Lacan further notes that "to love is, essentially, to wish to be loved" (Bowie, 1991, p. 103). For Lacan love entails only "an imaginary reciprocity" and mutuality, the "reciprocity between 'loving' and 'being loved'" that, along with the "fantasy of fusion" with the loved other mainly comprises the compelling illusion of love (Bowie, 1991, p. 103). Lacan rejects Freud and most other analysts who claim that love is the central clinical goal in psychoanalysis and, for that matter, the goal of life. Rather, he says that the aim of analysis is to reclaim the voice for one's desire by clarifying and making intelligible the familial experiences and knots, the governing signifiers, that have had such a powerful interpretive hold on one's way of being in the world. As far as I can tell, this may or may not lead to a greater capacity and actualization of love in one's way of being-in-the-world.

One of the limitations in the theorizing on love in Freud, Klein, Erikson, Kohut, and Lacan is that all of these theorists to some extent, treat the significant other reductively as a depersonalized love object, as a thing to be used for one's satisfaction. Even sophisticated relational theorists, like Jessica Benjamin, tend to view the other mainly as a source of reciprocal gratification of one's relational needs, which frequently results in two people in a doomed arrangement of mutually instrumental use (Benjamin, 1995).

Koheleth does not explain how he moved from the negative side of his ambivalence towards women, towards the positive one, but by the end of his book, he appears to have a degree of deep and abiding satisfaction with a woman, his version of love in the real world. Even without embracing a Levinasian shift to love, a being-for-the-other construct, psychoanalytic theorizing posits many ways to reach a mutually gratifying love relationship. So although we do not know how Koheleth transformed his ambivalence towards women, regarding them as toxic, to viewing them as nurturing and stable, we at least have some psychoanalytic conceptualizations to work with.

Case Vignette

Rolland, age 58, and ex patriate, lived in Colombia, South America, for the last 20 years. He came to me following the death of his mother in New York, a profound loss he claimed, as well as the fact that his three siblings had "turned against" him over the final care of his mother at her home (instead of being put in a nursing home). The three siblings, said Rolland, came together over the fact of their brother being perceived as the "favorite child" of his mother. This culminated in an incident two months before Rolland's mother had died, when Rolland's siblings called the police on him while he was taking care of his mother in her home (he slept there every day as well), claiming that he was psychologically abusing their mother. While the police turned up at his mother's house, Rolland was arrested and handcuffed, taken down to the station house, put in a holding pen, and ultimately freed for there was no compelling evidence against him. Subsequent to the arrest, Rolland had no contact with his siblings except through their lawyer. He had not seen his siblings for many years prior to his mother getting sick and rarely spoke to them during their adulthood. Rolland felt utterly betrayed by his siblings, often comparing them to Joseph's betrayal by his brothers who threw him into a pit and left him for dead. Rolland was deeply troubled by the fact that his siblings could be so mean and nasty and that he did not "see it coming." Rolland owned and operated a successful business and a French restaurant in Colombia. He said that he "loved" his work, he had no friends, and lived with a Colombia-born woman whom he was 30 years older than. She worked in a boutique selling high-end clothes while she went to university for a master's degree at night.

Rolland came to me during the final phase of his mother's life, about two years ago. I saw him twice a week with him complaining about feeling depressed and anxious and alienated from everyone. In fact, Roland often complained that he felt like "ET" being lost from his mothership, not really feeling that he was living an authentic life: "I don't know what I think, nor do I know what I am doing most of the day, just existing." Rolland complained that he was never sure he could trust his social perception, feeling somewhat like an imposter who had no psychological core.

Rolland was a very likeable and interesting man, very articulate and intelligent. He told me that since he lived in Colombia he had a "harem," that he visited every two weeks or so, in which he would "drink vodka, smoke weed, and have sex." Rolland especially enjoyed the threesomes he had with two women.

Rolland said that there was something of a quid pro quo between him and "his women." He gave them money towards their living expenses (they were financially needy and dependent), while he enjoyed being with these three women, whom he was 35 years older than. Rolland described his debauchery as the high point of his everyday existence. While Rolland engaged in his extracurricular sex with his harem, he also lived with a young woman named Suzannah whom he said he loved but was not willing or able to have sexual relations with. When I interpreted his sexual abstinence with Suzannah, he told me that he could not maintain an erection when with her and therefore avoided sexual contact on the rigorously sexual level. When I probed his sexual dysfunction, he said that his body "froze" when he thought of having sexual relations with Suzannah, though he emphasized that he "loved her," for she was a very nice person to talk to, and Suzannah appeared to take care of most of his emotional and practical needs. Rolland recognized that there was something disturbed and disturbing about him not being willing or able to have sex with Suzannah. He said he had tried to have sexual intercourse with her, but he froze and felt sick doing so.

Rolland also indicated that while Suzannah knew about his harem, she more or less accepted him having a need for sex with other women, though he only liked them, not loved them, he told me and Suzannah. Rolland had been briefly married when he was a younger man, having grown apart from his wife, also South American. He cheated on his wife and, subsequently, had two or three other serious relationships with South American women, in which he was chronically unfaithful. Rolland indicated that he also initially "loved" his wife and the women he had affairs with, though he soon grew bored with them. He was able to have episodic sex with all of these women but was frequently on the "hunt," as he characterized his behavior.

Rolland told me that he was worried and troubled that he was pushing age 60 and did not have a wife or children. He knew that his sexual interest would wane as he got a bit older and was deathly afraid of being alone for the rest of his life. On the other hand, Rolland said he was not willing and able to give up his harem, which as I said, was a source of great pleasure to him and was relatively harmless, he told me. Suzannah and his wife and other paramours all knew that he was episodically unfaithful, though they felt he was "good" to his wife and other women. Rolland had parted company with his wife and other two women due to irreconcilable differences, and the breakups were always amicable.

While I interpreted Rolland's sexual inhibition with his current girlfriend and debauchery with his harem in terms of his Mother-whore complex, none of my interpretations of him seeing Suzannah as the mother figure whom he wanted and needed to be close to as he was with his mother were successful. Nor were my interpretations of the fear of his cold and punitive father whom he feared would punish (and castrate) him for his sexual wishes towards his mother, a fear and panic that was evidenced by his freezing and feeling sick at the thought of sex with Suzannah. As Rolland told me, who would want to give up "drinking, weed and fucking, young women?" When I pointed out to Rolland that as he was nearing age 60 his sexual desire would wane, he told me that he could not imagine living in a traditional marital relationship, let alone having children, though he said that part of him wanted just that.

When I explored Rolland's relationship with Suzannah, he said that he did not know why she remained with him. Suzannah was beautiful, educated, and likeable, but she felt rejected by Rolland, though she never threatened to leave him in the lurch. Rolland reported feeling episodic guilt for his infidelity, though not so guilty that he stopped doing it. In addition to feeling episodic guilt, Rolland acknowledged that by not having sex with Suzannah, he in effect was withholding himself, an act of aggression towards her. A similar unconscious dynamic was in play with his mother, whom he withheld himself from, mainly because he could feel the hostility coming from his father and siblings.

Rolland also confessed that as with all of his choice of women, all very much younger South Americans, he felt a sense of "superiority" to them, them being much younger and coming from a third world country, as he called Colombia. Most importantly, Rolland said that he liked these women but did not love them, the way he did Suzannah. This sense of superiority over the young women gave us some understanding of his underlying insecurities such that he needed to be the one in control and have power over them. A power that was benignly exerted but hid the aggression towards the mother that was underneath it.

In the transference, Rolland tended to view me as a trusted confidante, going out of his way to maintain a cordial relationship. He did not experience me as judgmental or dismissive, but rather as a helpful doctor, as he called me, or the supportive mother. He has been able to recognize that he is secretly showing his aggression towards me and power over me by not letting me help him with his sexual inhibition with Suzannah. Roland also reported feeling somewhat guilty that he was the favorite son of his mother, although this honor came with alienation from his father and siblings, and the sense of entrapment by the mother that made him feel dependent and weak. This consideration may have contributed to his depressed feelings, which he felt as an adult from time to time. In addition, Rolland acknowledged that his detached and gruff father was jealous of his special status in regards to his mother, a kind of Oedipal victory.

Currently, Rolland says he is "stuck," as he calls it. He loves Suzannah but can't make love to her; he likes his harem, but he can't give it up as he ought to be able he said. Rolland has a nonexistent relationship with his siblings, who he says still hate him, and are contesting their mother's will giving Rolland the family home while his siblings divided the other monies (a fair deal said Rolland's lawyer). Rolland indicated that once the will is probated, he will not see or talk with his siblings though he expects them to appeal any decision that gives him the family home. Despite the harem, Rolland told me that he felt quite lonely at times and wished that he was willing and able to have a wife and children. "I am treading water," Rolland told me.

Notes

1 From a letter to Princess Maria Bonaparte in 1934, quoted in Steadman (1979).
2 I have, in part, based my summarizing comments on Robinson (1997).
3 Freud's heterosexual bias is here exemplified. The term "significant other" could be used as a replacement for "opposite sex."
4 I have liberally drawn from Evans for my summary of Lacan's theory, including using his Lacan quotations.
5 Briefly, according to Malcom Bowie (1991, p. 92), the Imaginary is the realm "of mirror images, identifications and reciprocities." The Symbolic "is the realm of language, the unconscious and the otherness" that stays other.
6 Sartre, too, claims that love can never really be other than the demand to be loved. This view follows from his questionable assumption that originally I am for-myself rather than for-the-Other.

8 Implications for Psychoanalysis

Koheleth puts forward a "religio-ethical standpoint" (Gordis, 1951, p. 80), a "religious consciousness" (Perry, 1993, p. 13) which characterizes his free associations on the meaning of human existence, the good that man can accomplish in life and the problematics of finding and/or creating a lasting sense of personal happiness.[1] Indeed, as Perry (1993) notes, Koheleth's "shopping list" of "dirty tricks," confronting humankind is clear and forceful: divine and human injustice, forgetfulness and death, the fruitlessness of our labor, the monotony of human history, and the repetitiveness of natural events (p. 3), and the fraught nature of human relationships.

Kugel (1996) provides an apt summary of Koheleth's "basic argument":

> Human existence, like so many things in the natural world (chapter 1), is round, circular; desires fit at one moment, when their time comes around, but not at another (chapter 3). Like a sphere, the whole life's surface cannot be described from any one angle; one must travel around it in order to account for all, and truths apparent from one standpoint prove to be *hebel* [vanity] from another.
>
> (pp. 259–260)

Koheleth's philosophy of life is in part rooted in the conviction that it is unwise, if not impossible to impose a comprehensive order and system, a worldview, on experience. For to do so is to do violence to experience, for example, reducing it to comfortable and banal formulas that do not do justice to the complexity, ambiguity, and contradictory character of experience. For Koheleth, the experience of life cannot be reduced to a system by means of moral principles since they collapse amid the anomalies of experience just as the attempt to reduce life to a system by means of theoretical ideas collapses as it tries to resolve the antinomies and paradoxes of existence (Guthrie and Motyer, 1970). In other words, as Levinas has suggested, we seem to have a basic tendency to totalize individual experience by assuming either that the world is entirely for us, or that the infinite (i.e., for Levinas, something-outside-everything, the Other or God) can actually be captured and

DOI: 10.4324/9781003652816-8

thus brought to reincorporate such pseudototalities into the infinite by the conclusion that God is to be feared (Perry, 1993). That is, God operates according to what appears to humans as an arbitrary and absolute determinism (e.g., we often feel like we live in an ethically uncaring universe).

While maintaining an antisystematicity assumption, Koheleth does nevertheless suggest that some attitudes toward life tend to be more useful than others. He thus offers some helpful, practical, experientially based attitudes towards existence that are strikingly compatible with a broadly conceived Freudian perspective. Both theoretical and clinical psychoanalysis can possibly benefit from being more cognizant of these attitudes as it both articulates its interesting and illuminating psychoanalytic narrative of the human condition and strives to help people achieve a greater degree of happiness amid their predicaments (Phillips, 1998). Indeed, Koheleth has a "harsh view of reality" that often resonates in the typical analysand in today's world (Murphy, 1992, p. xlix). In the spirit of Koheleth's dialogic, open, pluralistic, and non-authoritarian intellectual and spiritual approach to truth and reality (Perry, 1993), these attitudinal suggestions I describe represent some of the usable truths, as opposed to absolute Truths, that may be food for thought.

Throughout his experience-guided discourse, Koheleth asserts or implies that one must face the painful and distressing facts of life; that is, one must not continue to assert or accept as true that which does not hold up to critical evaluation, to the evidence, that to the orthodox theologians and priestly scribes of his day, it was believed that the righteous will be rewarded in this life and the wicked will be punished. However, experience indicated to him that this is frequently not the case. Moreover, Koheleth says that it is simply false that a commitment to wisdom, the striving after pleasure, or the hoarding of wealth and material possessions adds up to sustained, solid, let alone permanent happiness.

For the psychoanalyst, the idea that one must face facts and act accordingly is roughly similar to Freud's commitment to, and advocacy of, facing up to the hard truths about one's life even if the consequences are deeply disturbing. This idea speaks to what I believe is the heart of psychoanalysis. Continuing to assert so-called irrational and unreasonable convictions, to allow them to have a strong interpretive grip on one's outlook and behavior, is to succumb to neurosis. For example, the analysand who insists that his compulsive rituals and obsessive thinking actually protect him from external, real-life catastrophe is plainly not facing up to the evidence concerning the workings of the world. And the analysand who claims that having three consecutive marriages to men who turn out to be alcoholic is a sign of how defective contemporary men are in general, rather than accepting that it is she who unconsciously seeks out and chooses this type of man, is not facing up to the psychological evidence of her life. While no amount of so-called evidence and critical evaluation is a guarantee that has the Truth (since as I have said earlier, all evidence and facts are discourse specific, contestable, and can never be absolutely adjudicated); nevertheless, what Koheleth is pointing to is the importance of testing one's core convictions about one's life in terms of one's hard-earned experience, and have the courage and good sense to abandon claims that seem to go against the way the world hangs together.

A second attitude toward living that Koheleth articulates and that is fundamental to the psychoanalytic project is that one must learn to live with what cannot be altered and to submit to the inevitable (Scott, 1965). As Koheleth repeatedly notes, in a certain sense, "what is" cannot be changed by human efforts, and we do not know, and will never know, why God acts the way He does. In other words, the world keeps moving regardless of our wishes and our feeble efforts (relatively speaking) to intervene, and to understand why it moves in one way and not another is an eternal mystery. Whether we call it Providence, Fate, Luck, or the Reality principle, the point is the same, the need to accept life on its own terms since we are not in control of most things, let alone the really important things (e.g., "a time to be born and a time to die" – in both instances we have no choice in the matter).

In a similar way, the analysand who was abused or neglected as a child, or for that matter any patient who has suffered at the hands of his or her parents or from life's circumstances, needs to be able to accept that that which occurred is a harsh fact of their existence, an event that was out of their control and, in a certain sense, an affirmation of the irreversibility of lived time. For after all of the talking and working through of the personal meaning of the traumatic experiences, at the end of the day, the analysand has to accept that what was, was; it is a quirk of fate that he or she ended up in the circumstances they did (e.g., being born to abusive parents). We know that analysands tend to hold on to their pain and rage as they believe, usually insist, that it should have been otherwise and that they could have (should have) made it different. One way of understanding this is that they do not "fear God," as Koheleth calls it. That is, they are not conscious of His boundless and incomprehensible power (Gordis, 1951); they have not fully embraced their helplessness in the context of the arbitrary and absolute determinism of life. Without having internalized the notion that the world and its happenings remain fundamentally unknowable and uncontrollable, one will continue to hold on to one's pain and rage. That we cannot change what was means in a sense that we should avoid being fixed in a permanently intense retrospective consciousness, one that is in part driven by the angry claim that life is unfair. Narcissistic rage is "love outraged," said the Holocaust survivor analyst Henry Krystal. That is, where the expectation is to be loved, for example, to have a sense of self-worth and pride, one gets the opposite, traumatic assaults on one's self-esteem and self-concept (Krystal, 1988, p. 82).

Moreover, as we do not know what awaits us in the future, good or bad, we should surrender to our fate. *Amor fati*, love of fate, said Nietzsche. That is, it is prudent for us to make the most of the good times while we can and not be excessively troubled when things turn bad (Cohen, 1970). Embracing and loving everything that occurs in life, both positive and negative, as an essential aspect of one's existential odyssey.

As I have indicated, the logic of Koheleth's philosophy of life could well lead one to conclude that chronic despair is the only option. That is, as Koheleth describes it, given the fragility and impermanence of human accomplishments; the uncertainty and lack of control of our destiny; the impossibility of achieving true knowledge, understanding and insight into the world; and of course, inevitability of death, why bother living? And yet as I have earlier pointed out, Koheleth never advocates suicide nor despair, but rather insists that we are divinely obligated to make joy, including engaging in sensual pleasures, the goal of all our activities (Gordis, 1951). As Fox (2004) notes, "the heart" of Koheleth's insights is that we are not able to "know what will come to pass, so we must grasp whatever blessings the moment offers" (p. 47). Says Koheleth: "Therefore I praise joy, for there is no other good for man under the sun but to eat, drink, and be joyful and have this accompany him in his toil, during the days of his life, which God has given him beneath the sun" (Gordis, 1951, p. 174, 8:15). As Gordis indicates, Koheleth

> sets up the attainment of happiness as the goal of human striving, not merely because he loves life, but because he cannot have justice and wisdom [i.e., Truth]. Joy is the only purpose that he can find in a monotonous and meaningless world, in which all human values, such as wealth, piety, and ability, are vanity, where all men encounter the same fate and no progress is possible.
>
> (1951, p. 83)

In other words, for Koheleth, the only certainty that he has is that we have an intrinsic desire for happiness. Since God created humanity, He also created this desire, and therefore, Koheleth claims, that God's fundamental purpose for us is the deepening and expansion of our pleasures and the striving after happiness. To fail to obey this divine command is to be a sinner (Gordis, 1951, p. 115). I would add it also is foolish. For as Koheleth eloquently notes, it is the most sensible goal to enjoy life with all the relish one can muster, especially in one's youth, since we are vulnerable to the sudden and often cruel twists of fate, physical decline, and of course, death, the end of all activity, await us soon enough.

As the aforementioned suggests, Koheleth embodies what can be called "postmodern wisdom" (Bauman, 1993, p. 245). The brilliant Polish/British sociologist and philosopher Zygmunt Bauman explains what he means by the term. I quote the pertinent passage in full, for it conveys Koheleth's outlook rather well:

> What the postmodern mind is aware of is that there are problems in human and social life with no good solutions, twisted trajectories that cannot be

> straightened up, ambivalences that are more than linguistic blunders yelling to be corrected, doubts which cannot be legislated out of existence, moral agonies which no reason-directed recipes can soothe, let alone cure. The postmodern mind does not expect any more to find the all-embracing, total and ultimate formula of life without ambiguity, risk, dangers and error, and is deeply suspicious of any voice that promises otherwise.

That is, says Bauman:

> The postmodern mind is aware that each local, specialized and focused treatment, effective or not when measured by its ostensive target, spoils as much as, if not more than, it repairs. The postmodern mind is reconciled to the idea that the messiness of the human predicament is here to stay. That is, in the broadest outlines, what can be called postmodern wisdom.
>
> (1993, p. 245)

What Does Koheleth Base His Postmodern Wisdom On?

Fox (2004) has aptly pointed out that Koheleth's fundamental grievance is the irrationality of the world and how to navigate one's existential odyssey within this challenging context. That is, life's absurdities frustrate the rational mind and compromise a person's ability to effectively manage the world. As we cannot discern what will transpire so we must seize whatever blessings the moment provides (pp. xxx, xvii, 47). Paraphrasing Koheleth, 8:15, "Eat, drink, and be merry because tomorrow we die." Given the finite and transitory nature of life, it is essential that we enjoy ourselves with the fullness of our whole being. As Seow points out, "The point of the whole book" of Ecclesiastes "as a whole is that all people, male and female, are under this burden of toil – not only men." By toil is meant the "physical or intellectual struggle to achieve some end or other" (Seow, 1997, pp. x, 48). For Koheleth, the end is joy and happiness.

I have suggested that Koheleth advocates the importance of a love relationship (of any persuasion, in my view), and zestful and purposeful activity to attaining a degree of happiness. No psychoanalyst would disagree with this. However, what Koheleth adds here is rarely emphasized in the psychoanalytic narrative yet is an insight that can only heighten the satisfaction associated with love and purposeful activity. Following Freud, I am referring to the fact that the enjoyment of these experiences is enhanced by a greater mindfulness of the transitoriness of life. Moreover, it is this sense of resignation in the face of the brevity of life, in the face of a life's all-too-frequent frustration and harshness, that makes these experiences that much more enjoyable and lasting. Such an attitude also fosters one of the most underrated sensibilities in the modern secular world, a sensibility that religious traditions have emphasized as fundamental to attaining a degree of happiness, a sense of gratitude for what one has. For Koheleth, as I have said, a certain downsizing of one's narcissism is a prerequisite for even episodic and praiseworthy pleasure, let alone a more solid and lasting sense of happiness.

In contrast, Koheleth mocks the masses of people who choose to live their lives in a way that is not mindful of the tragic (or tragicomic) character as described throughout this book. These are the narcissists and those, for example, who are driven by envy and greed, who do not embrace with melancholic resignation (though without despair), the absolute limitations on existence, and who have not cultivated a sense of gratitude for that which they do have. Such people insist that they are masters of their own destiny, that through seeking and attaining more and more acquisitions they will be forever safe and happy. As psychoanalyst Erich Fromm (1994) noted in *Escape of Freedom*, "Greed is a bottomless pit which exhausts the person in an endless effort to satisfy the need without ever reaching satisfaction" (p. 79). Fromm's quote suggests that greed is not merely a desire for more and more, but a basic fault that leads to an endless cycle of unhappiness and emotional exhaustion.

Finally, I have attempted to illustrate in this book some of the brilliant and profound insights about the human condition that are embodied in the ethical wisdom of Koheleth and may, in some form, enhance theoretical and clinical psychoanalysis, conceived in this book as a "practice of the self." Most important, Koheleth advocates resignation without despair, that is, cultivating an inner attitude toward life that strives to transcend the tragic limitations and pangs and sorrows of existence through a frank and courageous acceptance that they cannot be transformed. For Koheleth this promotes dedicating oneself to striving after joy in life, not so much for the reasons the idealistic pious believe, because it is a gift from God to be treasured, but because the search for joy is the only sensible goal, considering the frustrating, tragic, and fundamentally futile nature of existence. Freud probably saw life in a similar way when he famously wrote that the purpose of psychoanalysis was to transform "hysterical [neurotic] misery into common unhappiness" (Breuer and Freud, 1893–1895, p. 305).

Note

1 I have in part drawn from Marcus (2003) in this conclusion.

References

Akhtar, S. (2009). *Comprehensive Dictionary of Psychoanalysis*. London: Karnac Books.

Alford, C.F. (1998). Melanie Klein and the nature of good and evil. In Marcus, P., and Rosenberg, A. (eds.), *Psychoanalytic Versions of the Human Condition, Philosophies of Life and Their Impact on Practice*. New York: New York University Press, 118–139.

Allen, R.E. (ed.) (1990). *The Concise Oxford Dictionary*. Oxford: Clarendon Press, 708.

Allport, G.W. (1937). *Personality: A Psychological Interpretation*. New York: Holt.

Alter, R. (2010). *The Wisdom Books: Job, Proverbs, and Ecclesiastes*. New York: W.W. Norton.

Ambrose, D. (2022). Wisdom and social policy. In Sternberg, R.J., and Gluck, J. (eds.), *The Psychology of Wisdom. An Introduction*. Cambridge: Cambridge University Press, 245–261.

Bartholomew, C.G. (2009). *Ecclesiastes*. Grand Rapids, MI: Baker Publishing Group.

Bass, A. (1998). Sigmund Freud. The question of a Weltanschauung and of defense. In Marcus, P., and Rosenberg, A. (eds.), *Psychoanalytic Versions of the Human Condition: Philosophies of Life and Their Impact on Practice*. New York: New York University Press, 412–446.

Bauman, Z. (1993). *Postmodern Ethics*. Oxford: Blackwell.

Becker, E. (1969). *Angel in Armor: A Post-Freudian Perspective on the Nature of Man*. New York: Braziller.

Bellah, R.N., Madsen, R., Swidler, A., and Tipton, S.M. (1986). *Habits of the Heart: Individuation and Commitment in American Life*. New York: Harper and Row.

Benjamin, J. (1995). An outline of intersubjectivity: The development of mutual recognition. *Psychoanalytic Psychology* 7: 33–46.

Berg, J.M., Grant, A.G., and Johnson, V. (2010). When callings are calling: Crafting work and leisure in pursuit of unanswered occupational callings. *Organization Sciences* 21(5): 973–994.

Berger, P.L. (1997). *Redeeming Laughter. The Comic Dimension of Human Experience*. Berlin: Walter De Gruyter.

Bergmann, M.S. (1987). *The Anatomy of Loving: The Story of Man's Quest to Know What Love Is*. New York: Fawcett Columbine.

Blum, H.P. (1997). Psychoanalysis and playful work. In Socarides, C.W., and Kramer, S. (eds.), *Work and Its Inhibitions: Psychoanalytic Essays*. Madison, WI: International University Press, 19–34.

Bowie, M. (1991). *Lacan*. London: Fontana Press.

Breuer, J., and Freud, S. (1893–1895). Studies on hysteria. In Strachey, J. (ed.), *Standard Edition of the Complete Psychological Works of Sigmund Freud*, Volume 2. London: Hogarth Press and the Institute of Psycho-Analysis, 1953–1974, 1–323.

Carr, A. (2022). *Positive Psychology. The Science of Wellbeing and Human Strengths*. 3rd edition. London: Routledge.

Cohen, A. (ed.) (1970). *The Five Megillot*. London: Soncino Press.

Compton, W.C., and Hoffman, E. (2020). *Positive Psychology. The Science of Happiness and Flourishing*. Los Angeles, CA: Sage.

Crenshaw, J.L. (1987). *Ecclesiastes. A Commentary*. Philadelphia, PA: Westminster Press.

Csikszentmihalyi, M. (1975). Play and intrinsic rewards. *Journal of Humanistic Psychology* 15: 41–63.

Erikson, E.H. (1950). *Childhood and Society*. 2nd edition. New York: W.W. Norton.

Erikson, E.H. (1959). Identity and the life cycle. *Psychological Issues* 1: 1–173.

Erikson, E.H. (1964). *Insight and Responsibility*. New York: W.W. Norton.

Erikson, E.H. (1982). *The Life Cycle Completed*. New York: W.W. Norton.

Erikson, E.H., Erikson, J.M., and Kivnick, H.Q. (1986). *Vital Involvement in Old Age. The Experience of Old Age in Our Time*. New York: W.W. Norton.

Evans, D. (1996). *An Introductory Dictionary of Lacanian Psychoanalysis*. London: Routledge.

Fackenheim, E. (1996). *Jewish Philosophers and Jewish Philosophy* (M.L. Morgan, ed.). Bloomington, IN: Indiana University Press.

Fadiman, C., and Brand, A. (eds.) (1985). *Bartlette Book of Anecdotes*. New York: Little, Brown & Co.

Ferry, L. (2005). *What Is the Good Life* (L.G. Cochrone, trans.). Chicago, IL: University of Chicago Press.

Fine, R. (1979). *History of Psychoanalysis*. New York: Columbia University Press.

Foucault, M. (1989). The ethics of the concern for self as a practice of freedom. In S. Lotringer (ed.), *Foucault Live: Collected Interviews, 1961–1984*. New York: Semiotexte, 432–449.

Fox, M.V. (1999). *A Time to Tear Down and a Time to Build Up: A Rereading of Ecclesiastes*. Eugene: Wipf & Stock Publishers.

Fox, M.V. (2004). *Ecclesiastes*. Philadelphia, PA: Jewish Publication Society.

Freud, S. (1905/1953). Three essays on the theory of sexuality. In Strachey, J. (ed. and trans.), *Standard Edition of the Complete Psychological Works of Sigmund Freud*, Volume 7. London: Hogarth Press, 130–245.

Freud, S. (1910/1963). *Psychoanalysis and Faith. The Letters of Sigmund Freud and Oskar Pfister* (H. Meng and E.L. Feder, eds., E. Mosbacher, trans.). London: Hogarth Press.

Freud, S. (1912/1957). On the universal tendency to debasement in the sphere of love. In Strachey, J. (ed. and trans.), *Standard Edition of the Complete*

Psychological Works of Sigmund Freud, Volume 11. London: Hogarth Press, 179–190.

Freud, S. (1915/1914). Observations on transference-love. Further recommendations on the technique of psycho-analysis. In Strachey, J. (ed. and trans.), *Standard Edition of the Complete Psychological Works of Sigmund Freud*, Volume 12. London: Hogarth Press, 1958, 159–171.

Freud, S. (1915/1916). On transience. In Strachey, J. (ed. and trans.), *Standard Edition of the Complete Psychological Works of Sigmund Freud*, Volume 14. London: Hogarth Press, 305–307.

Freud, S. (1916–1917/1961). Introductory lectures on psycho-analysis. In Strachey, J. (ed. and trans.), *Standard Edition of the Complete Psychological Works of Sigmund Freud*, Volumes 15 and 16. London: Hogarth Press.

Freud, S. (1927/1961). The future of illusion. In Strachey, J. (ed. and trans.), *Standard Edition of the Complete Psychological Works of Sigmund Freud*, Volume 21. London: Hogarth Press, 5–56.

Freud, S. (1930/1961). *Civilization and Its Discontents*. In Strachey, J. (ed. and trans.), *Standard Edition of the Complete Psychological Works of Sigmund Freud*, Volume 21. London: Hogarth Press, 57–145.

Freud, S. (1937/1961). *Letters of Sigmund Freud* (E.L. Freud, ed.). New York: Basic Books.

Fromm, E. (1994). *Escape from Freedom*. New York: Holt Paperbacks.

Fryer, D.R. (2004). *The Intervention of the Other*. New York: Other Press.

Gedo, J.E. (1997). In praise of leisure. In Socarides, C.W., and Kramer, S. (eds.), *Work and Its Inhibitions: Psychoanalytic Essays*. Madison: International University Press, 133–141.

Gibson, D. (2017). *Living Life Backwards. How Ecclesiastes Teaches Us to Live in Light of the End*. Wheaton: Crossway.

Ginsberg, H.L. (1969). *The Five Megilloth and Jonah*. Philadelphia, PA: Jewish Publication Society.

Gordis, R. (trans. and commentator) (1951). *Koheleth – The Man and His World*. New York: Jewish Theological Seminary of America.

Guthrie, D., and Motyer, J.A. (eds.) (1970). *The New Bible Commentary, Revised*. Grand Rapids, MI: Eerdmans Publishing Company.

Hadot, P. (1997). *Philosophy as a Way of Life*. Oxford: Blackwell.

Hale, N.G. (ed.). (1971). *James Jackson Putnam and Psychoanalysis. Letters Between Putnam and Sigmund Freud, Ernest Jones, William James, Sandor Ferenczi and Morton Price. 1877–1917* (J.B. Heller, trans.). Cambridge: Cambridge University Press.

Heim, K.M. (2019). *Ecclesiastes*. Downers Grove: IVP Academic.

Heim, K.M. (2025). Personal communication.

Johnson, B., VanderWeele, T.J., and Case, B. (2025). Turns out, G.D.P. doesn't buy happiness, opinion section. *New York Times*, 3 May, p. A26.

Jones, E. (1953–1957). *The Life and Work of Sigmund Freud*, 3 Volumes. New York: Basic Books.

Jordan, J. (2005). The quest for wisdom in adulthood. A psychological perspective. In Sternberg, R.J., and Jordan, J.A. (eds.), *Handbook of Wisdom. Psychological Perspectives*. Cambridge: Cambridge University Press, 160–188.

Kahana, R. (1978). The Psychoanalysis in Later Life: Discussion. *Journal of Geriatric Psychiatry* 11: 37–49.

Keynes, W. (2019). *An Obituary for "Wisdom Literature": The Birth, Death, and Intertextual Reintegration of a Biblical Corpus.* Oxford: Oxford University Press.

Kohut, H. (1984). *How Does Analysis Cure?* Chicago, IL: University of Chicago Press.

Koltko-Rivera, M.E. (2004). The psychology of worldviews. *Review of General Psychology* 8(1): 3–58.

Krystal, H. (1988). *Integration and Self-Healing: Affect, Healing and Alexithymia.* London: Routledge.

Kugel, J.L. (1996). Ecclesiastes. In Achtemeir, P.J. (ed.), *Bible Dictionary*, Revised edition. San Francisco, CA: Harper, 258–260.

Kunzmann, U., and Baltes, P.B. (2005). The psychology of wisdom. Theoretical and empirical challenges. In Sternberg, R.J., and Jordan, J. A. (eds.), *Handbook of Wisdom. Psychological Perspectives*. Cambridge: Cambridge University Press, 110–135.

Kupperman, J.J. (2005). Morality, ethics, and wisdom. In Sternberg, R.J., and Jordan, J. (eds.), *A Handbook of Wisdom. Psychological Perspectives.* Cambridge: Cambridge University Press, 245–271.

Lazari-Radek, K., and Singer, P. (2025). The lesson from a Nobel Laureate's chosen death. *New York Times*, Opinion Section, 20 April, p. 8.

Levinas, E. (1969). *Totality and Infinity: An Essay on Exteriority* (A. Lingis, trans.). Pittsburgh, PA: Duquesne University Press.

Levinas, E. (1981). *Otherwise Than Being or Beyond Essence* (A. Lingis, trans.). The Hague; Boston, MA; London: Nijhoff (Kluwer).

Levinas, E. (1987). *The Levinas Reader* (S. Hand, trans.). Oxford: Basil Blackwell Publishing.

Levinas, E. (1989). *Difficult Freedom: Essays on Judaism* (S. Hand, ed.). Baltimore, MD: Johns Hopkins University Press.

Lifton, R.J. (1976). *The Life of the Self: Toward a New Psychology*. New York: Basic Books.

Liu, X. (1990). Taoism. In Sharma, A. (ed.), *Our Religions*. San Francisco, CA: Harper.

Loader, J.A. (1986). *Ecclesiastes. A Practical Commentary*. Grand Rapids, MI: William B. Eerdmans Publishing Company.

Lohfink, N. (2003). *Qoheleth. A Continental Commentary* (S. McEvenue, trans.). Minneapolis, MN: Fortress Press.

Longman III, T. (1998). *The Book of Ecclesiastes*. Grand Rapids, MI: William B. Eerdmans Publishing Company.

Marcus, P. (2003). *Ancient Religious Wisdom, Spirituality and Psychoanalysis*. Westport, CT: Praeger.

Marcus, P. (2013). *How to Laugh Your Way Through Life*. London: Karnac Books.

Marcus, P., and Rosenberg, A. (eds.) (1998). *Psychoanalytic Versions of the Human Condition. Philosophies of Life and Their Impact on Practice.* New York: New York University Press.

Maxwell, N. (2007). From knowledge to wisdom: The need for an academic revolution. *London Review of Education* 5(2): 97–115.
McGuire, W. (ed.). (1974). *The Freud/Jung letters*. Princeton, NJ: Princeton University Press.
McIntire, D.C. (2020). *Catching the Wind. A Guide to Interpreting Ecclesiastes*. Murrells Inlet: Covenant Books.
Monte, C. (1980). *Beneath the Mask. An Introduction to Theories of Personality*. 2nd edition. New York: Holt, Rineheart and Winston.
Moore, B.E., and Fine, B.D. (eds.) (1990). *Psychoanalytic Terms and Concepts*. New Haven, CT: American Psychoanalytic Association and Yale University Press.
Murphy, R. (1992). *Ecclesiastes. Word Biblical Commentary*. Grand Rapids, MI: Zonderman Academic.
Neff, W.S. (1965). Psychoanalytic conceptions of the meaning of work. *Psychiatry* 28(4): 324–333.
Osbeck, L.M., and Robinson, D.N. (2005). Philosophical theories of wisdom. In Sternberg, R.J., and Jordan, J.A. (Eds.), *Handbook of Wisdom. Psychological Perspectives*. Cambridge: Cambridge University Press, 61–83.
Patterson, E.M. (1984). The Holocaust as sin: Requirements in psychoanalytic theory for human evil and mature morality. In Luel, S.A., and Marcus, P. (eds.), *Psychoanalytic Reflections on the Holocaust: Selected Essays*. New York: University of Denver and KTAV, 70–91.
Perry, T.A. (1993). *Dialogues with Kohelet. The Book of Ecclesiastes*. University Park, PA: Pennsylvania State University Press.
Person, E.S., Cooper, A.M., and Gabbard, G.O. (eds.) (2005). *Textbook of Psychoanalysis*. Washington, DC: American Psychiatric Publishing.
Peterson, C., and Seligman, M.E. (2004). *Character Strengths and Virtues. A Handbook and Classification*. Oxford University Press.
Phillips, A. (1998). Paging Dr. Freud. *New York Times Book Review*, 7 June, p. 24.
Phillips, A. (2021). *The Cure for Psychoanalysis*. London: Confer Books.
Razinsky, L. (2015). On time, transience and literary creation: Freud and Rilke a century ago. *Modern Language Studies* 51(4): 464–478.
Reik, T. (1983). *Listening with the Third Ear*. New York: Farrar, Straus and Giroux.
Richardson, M.J., and Pasupathi, M. (2005). *Handbook of Wisdom. Psychological Perspectives* (R.J. Sternberg and J.A. Jordan, eds.). Cambridge: Cambridge University Press, 139–159.
Robinson, D.N. (1997). *The Great Ideas of Philosophy*, Part 2. Chantilly, VA: The Teaching Company, Course Outline, 12–15.
Root, E.T. (1889). Ecclesiastes considered psychologically. *Old and New Testament Student* 93: 138–142.
Rotenstreich, N. (1968). *Jewish Philosophy in Modern Times. From Mendelssohn to Rosenzweig*. New York: Holt, Rinehart and Winston.
Rycroft, C. (1995). *Dictionary of Psychoanalysis*. London: Penguin Books.
Ryken, P.G. (2015). *Why Everything Matters. The Gospel in Ecclesiastes*. Scotland: Christian Focus Publications.

Sachs, J. (2025a). Shabbat announcements. *Great Neck Synagogue*, 12 April, pp. 1–2.

Sachs, J. (2025b). Shabbat announcements. *Great Neck Synagogue*, 5 April, pp. 1–2.

Sachs, J. (2025c). Shabbat announcements. *Great Neck Synagogue*, 19 April, pp. 1–2.

Scott, R.B.Y. (ed.). (1965). *The Anchor Bible: Proverbs: Ecclesiastes*. Garden City: Double Day and Company.

Seow, C.L. (1997). *Ecclesiastes. A New Translation with Introduction and Commentary*. New Haven, CT: Yale University Press.

Shields, M.A. (2006). *The End of Wisdom. A Reappraisal of the Historical and Canonical Function of Ecclesiastes*. Winona Lake: Eisenbrauns.

Snowdon, D.A. (2002). *Aging with Grace: What the Nun Study Teaches Us About Living Longer, Healthier and More Meaningful Lives*. New York: Bantam.

Solms, M. (2024). Conversation with Mark Solms. *Psychoanalytic Review* 111(4): 384–412.

Solomon, J.L., Marshall, P., and Gardner, H. (2005). Crossing boundaries to generative wisdom. In Sternberg, R.J., and Jordan, J.A. (eds.), *Handbook of Wisdom. Psychological Perspectives*, Cambridge: Cambridge University Press, 272–296.

Staudinger, U.M., Dorner, J., and Mickler, C. (2005). Wisdom and personality. In Sternberg, R.J., and Jordan, J.A. (eds.), *Handbook of Wisdom. Psychological Perspectives*. Cambridge: Cambridge University Press, 191–219.

Steadman, R. (1979). *Sigmund Freud.* New York: Paddington Press.

Sternberg, R.J., and Gluck, J. (2022). Introduction. What is wisdom and why Is it important. In Sternberg, R.J., and Gluck, J. (eds.), *The Psychology of Wisdom. An Introduction*. Cambridge: Cambridge University Press, 3–14.

The New York Times Magazine (2025). The Happiness Issue. 4 May.

Watson, B. (1958). *The Complete Works of Chuang Tzu*. New York: Columbia University Press.

Weeks, S. (2020). *A Critical and Exegetical Commentary on Ecclesiastes, Volume 1: Introduction and Commentary on Ecclesiastes 1.1–5.6*. London: T&T Clark.

Weinstein, F. (1990). *History and Theory After the Fall*. Chicago, IL: University of Chicago Press.

Zimmermann, F. (1973). *The Inner World of Qohelet*. New York: KTAV.

Zlotowitz, M. (1994). *Koheles: Ecclesiastes: A New Translation with Commentary Anthologized from the Talmudic, Midrashic and Rabbinic Sources*. Brooklyn, NY: Mesorah Publications.

Internet Sources

https://www.freud.org.uk › Blog Accessed 25 February 2025.

www.quoteworld.org › Mark Twain Accessed 1 March 2025.

https://www.sefaria.org ›... › Daf 13b › Line 11 Accessed 20 February 2025.

Index

absurd 12, 14, 33–34, 36, 41, 81
acceptance 3, 33, 37–39, 41, 82
addiction 45, 48
affluence (abundance) 19
ageing 29–30, 51
aggression 55, 71, 75–76
Akhtar, S. 38, 61
alcohol 48, 78
Aleichem, Sholom 14
Alford, C.F. 71
Alter, R. 2, 6–7, 9, 25
ambiguity 4–5, 7–9, 58, 77, 81
ambivalence 5, 7, 9, 46, 49, 58, 66, 69, 71, 73, 81
Ambrose, D. 32
anhedonia (inability to experience pleasure) 45, 62
Aristotle 24–25, 69
authority 11, 22, 25

baraita 43n4
Bartholomew, C.G. 2, 6n7, 9, 25, 38–39
Bass, A. 8
Bauman, Z. 80–81
behavior: acceptable/unacceptable 8, 51, 58, 67, 78; hedonic 45; motivation of 15, 21, 33, 38, 47; transforming 5
beliefs (core) 1–3, 8
Bellah, R.N. (et al 1986) 60–61, 63n3
Benjamin, J. 73
Berger, P.L. 13–14
Bonaparte, Marie 36, 66, 76n1
Bowie, M 76n5
burnout 57

carpe diem 31n5, 46, 49, 71
Carr, S. 34, 37
civilization 2, 37, 58, 60, 69, 72
cognition 11, 34
Cohen, A. 31n8
companionship 56, 64, 66
Compton, W.C. 47
conservative 3, 11, 39
contemporary: life 2; views 37, 51, 78
contradiction 5, 7–9, 11, 18, 26, 39, 77
Crenshaw, J.L. 2, 9, 33
Csikszentmihalyi, M. 56
cyclicality 17
cynicism 13, 23, 42, 66

death: certainty of 4, 10, 30, 38, 50, 80; day of 24; fear of 37–39; meaning of 13, 17, 27–28
depression 10, 31n4, 36, 45, 49, 52, 61, 63, 74, 76
despair 4, 37–40, 48, 80, 82
diligence 23, 51
drugs, use of 48, 61, 75

Ecclesiastes: fictional royal autobiography 15n7; poetic perceptiveness 2, 30; political satire 1, 13; voices of 6n7, 17; writer of 2–3, 6n1; *see also* Koheleth
ego: consciousness 32; development of 32, 37; integrity 37–39; toxic 31, 51; *see also* narcissism
emotional: bond 70, 74; stability 33; suffering 57, 65, 82; trials 21, 30
envy 12, 31n4, 50–51, 55, 82
Erikson, E. 5, 36–39, 41, 72
Eros 37, 58, 72
Evans, D. 73, 76n4
excess, danger of 6n6
expectation 24, 52–53, 79

Fackenheim, E.L. 15n2
failure, feelings of 41, 61
faith: lack of 64; person of 1, 4, 10, 30, 43, 51
fame 22, 51, 56–57, 66
family: life 21, 47; nuclear 61; relationships 40, 52, 61, 72–76
fatalism 18, 49
fate 12–13, 24, 27, 80; amor fati (love of fate) 79
Fertile Crescent 3
fetishization 50–51, 62
financial: consultant 61; needs 74; success 60, 6262
Fine, R. 70
Fleiss, W. 37
folly 10, 12, 19, 21, 25, 28, 35–36, 44; *see also* wickedness
fool 10, 19, 22–23, 25, 28, 36, 55–56
Foucault, M. 4
Fox, M.V. 2, 6n7, 7, 9, 13, 20, 25, 33, 36, 45–46, 55–56, 64–65, 80–81
Franklin, B. 41
freedom 5, 18, 33, 44, 63n1
Freud, S. 4–5, 7–8, 11–13, 15, 18, 21–22, 33, 36–37, 39
friendship 69
Fromm. E. 82
futility: of life 5, 24, 33, 39, 66; of wisdom 5, 7; of work 5, 12, 68

Gedo, J.E. 63n1
Ginsberg, H.L. 31n8, 32, 71
God: Commandments of 3, 6, 11, 25, 28, 30, 33, 42, 68; favour of 19; fear of/reverence for 11, 22, 25, 28, 43n3, 78; gifts of 15, 21, 46; name of 9; omnipotence of 9, 30; power of 22; purpose of 15, 16n4; relationship with 14–15; will of 18, 23
golden mean 3, 24–25
Gordis, R. 1–2, 5, 7, 11, 13, 17, 28, 30n1, 39, 43n1, 43n7, 55, 64, 80
Grandma Moses 22, 31n4, 43, 50, 52, 71, 81–82
gratitude 22, 31n4, 43, 50, 52, 71, 81–82
greed 23, 50–51, 82

Hadot, P. 4
happiness: personal 1, 4, 77; quest for 21, 25; research 6n3
harshness 18, 21, 27, 50, 78–79, 81
Hebrew Bible 1, 3
hedonism: futility of 5, 44; sub-species of (Epicureanism) 44–45
Heim, K.M. 1–2, 7, 13, 31n8, 33, 42, 43n1, 46, 54n1
hevel (Hebrew word, primarily found in the Book of Ecclesiastes, which generally translates to "vanity," "futility," or "meaninglessness"-Google translate) 33, 43n2
Hoffman, E. 47
hostility 58, 75
human: accomplishments 18, 50, 67–68, 80; actions, preordained 10, 18–19, 23–24; consciousness 8, 45, 51–52, 77, 79; desires 10, 29, 45–46, 54, 67, 77; existence 3–4, 13, 77; suffering 4, 12–13, 21, 23, 40, 46, 55–56, 65

humanism 5
humanity 2, 23, 33, 58, 69, 80
humility 34
humor 13–14, 33

identity 4–5, 32, 42, 60–61, 72
illusion 15, 43n7, 73
injustice 11, 77
insecurity 57
integrity 37–39, 41
irony 1, 13–15, 39, 54
irrationality 36, 81

Jerusalem 2, 6n7, 17, 35, 44
Job 3, 9
joy: of creation 21, 55; the divine imperative 28; house of 24; striving for 4, 19, 39
justice 10–11, 14–15, 21–22, 27, 77, 80

Kahana, R. 39
Kahneman, D. 43n8
Kant, I. 45
Keynes, W. 6n5
King David 3, 17
Klein, M. 5, 71, 73
knowledge: of death 4, 10, 16n8, 30, 38, 50; limitations of 18–19; wisdom in 32, 34–35, 42
Koheleth (Hebrew name for the author of the Book of Ecclesiastes): neurotic analysand 9; outlook on life 1, 5, 13, 18, 38–39, 48, 80; teacher of wisdom or comic? 2–3, 6n2, 12–13; teacher/thinker 12
Kohut, H. 5, 72–73
Koltko-Rivera, M.E. 8
Krystal, H. 79
Kugel, J.L. 77

labour/labor: life's activities 56 (*see also* work); reward 19, 21, 44, 55–56
Lacan, J. 5, 72–73, 76n4
language 2, 6n4, 11, 49, 51–52, 71, 76n5
laziness 19, 21, 28
Levinas, E. 5, 45, 51, 66, 68
libido 36, 59, 71
life: absurdity of 33; conduct 1–2, 18, 59, 61; control, feeling out of 40, 52; development 34, 37–38, 41, 47, 61, 72; meaning of 14, 23, 36–37, 49, 80; mystery of 10, 18, 24, 33, 35; pleasures of 13, 19, 21, 45–46, 66, 68; purpose 14–15, 20, 28, 36, 42, 46, 68, 80; seasons of 13, 20, 38, 79; transitoriness of 50, 81
Lifton, R. J. 10
limitations 4, 6n4, 7, 18, 48, 50, 67, 73, 82
Liu, X. 20
Loader, J.A. 9, 28
Lohfink, N. 1
lonely 62, 76
Longman III, T. 2, 12–13, 16n4, 16n8
love: brotherly 69; capacity to 5, 12, 53, 63n1, 70, 73; forms of 69–70; futility of 5, 64; need for 60, 71; perfected 69; psychoanalytical view 69–71; relationship 49, 64–66, 72–73, 81

madness 27, 35, 43n6
Marcus, P. 82n1
marriage: infidelity 52–53, 75; life-partner 40, 67–68; unfulfilling 39, 45–46, 52–54, 61
material pleasures 19, 25; *see also* affluence
Maxwell, N. 43n5
meaning: maintenance 11; search for 1, 5, 12, 14–15, 18, 23, 36–37, 77
meaningless 12, 18, 45, 51, 80
Meltzer, D. 71
Melville, Herman *("Moby Dick")* 1
memory 13
Mill, John Stuart 45
mindfulness 50, 68, 81

money, love of 23, 50, 62
Monte, C. 37
mortality saliency 10, 12–13, 30, 39
Mother Theresa 41
motivation 10, 12, 22, 32, 45, 49, 57, 60, 91
mourn/mourning 13, 20, 24, 29, 48–49, 58, 63
Murphy, R. 1–2, 7
mystery of the world 10, 24, 33, 35, 79

narcissism 20, 23, 50–51, 70, 82
narrative 2, 4–5, 9, 30, 32, 49, 78
narrator 6n7, 17, 25, 42
Neff, W.S. 58
negative emotions 33, 42, 45
neglect 45, 57, 79
neurosis 11, 63n2, 78

obligations 3, 22, 45, 52, 58
obsession 16n8, 23, 62, 78
Old Testament traditions 9
optimism 3, 5, 18, 41
orthodox 3–4, 42, 68, 78

parody 1, 13
Perry, T.A. 1–2, 17, 33, 51, 77
Person, E.S. (et al 2021) 55
pessimism 3, 5, 11, 16n7, 17–18, 48, 67
Pfister, O. 67
piety 22, 80
pleasure: essence of 45, 47; pursuit of 44, 49
pleasure-seeking 5, 37, 44–45, 47–49
pleasure-unpleasure principle 47, 59
poor man 22–23, 28, 36, 56
positive emotions 31n4, 33, 48
pride 39, 79
Proverbs, Book of 3, 12
psychoanalysis: spiritual exercise 4–5; use of 5, 8
purity 65

Razinsky, L. 54n2
reality principle 32, 47, 59–60, 79
reason: use of 3–4; voice of 12
reasoning 11, 32, 34
Reik, T. 52
rejoice 6, 19, 21, 29, 44, 68
relationship: dialectic 9, 11, 60; love 49, 64–66, 72–73, 81; *see also* marriage
religion 15, 38
resignation without despair 4, 11, 14, 42, 50, 81–82
responsible pleasure 5, 47, 49
retribution 26–27, 42
reverence 9, 22, 25
reward 13, 19, 21, 26–27, 44, 56, 61, 65, 78
rivalry 12, 21, 55
Robinson, D.N. 76n2
Rycroft, C. 48

Sachs, J. 31n4, 43n2, 46
satisfaction: lasting 12, 18, 73; personal 18, 59, 65, 72, 82
Scott, R.B.Y. 3
self, sense of 50, 60, 72, 79
self-indulgence 45
self-love 66
selfobject 72
self-reflection 10
self-study 7
self-transcendence 5, 38, 43
self-transformation 2, 5, 52
self-understanding 5
sensual pleasure 47, 49, 65, 69, 80
Seow 2–3, 13, 15n1, 18, 22, 33, 41–42, 81
sexual: desire 66, 75; dysfunction 74; relations 61, 74
social: connectivity 6n3; paradigm 4, 34; status 23, 28, 36; structure 11
Solms, M. 18
Solomon (King) 3, 6n7, 17, 35, 42
spirituality 33, 38
spiritual traveler 7
state of mind 2, 23
Steadman, R. 76n1
Sternberg, R.J. 32
stress 57, 59
success 60, 62–63; desire for 22–23, 60; lack of 62; path to 28, 31n4, 48

suicide 34, 43n8, 80
sun, nothing new under 17, 39, 43
superiority, sense of 75–76
support 2, 28, 52, 57, 60–61, 63, 68, 72
synagogue 3, 6n7

Tao/Taoism 20
tension 11, 47
Thanatos 37, 72
theologians 3, 8, 78
theology 15
toil (work) 12, 17, 19–21, 27, 41, 46, 55, 65, 80–81
tragicomic outlook 13–14, 42
transcendence 10–11, 16n3, 38, 51; *see also* self-transcendence
transience 16n7, 22, 48–49
translation 1–2, 6n4, 37
truth 5; love of 11, 57; search for 11, 18, 35; usable 11, 78
Twain, M. 58

unpleasure 47, 59

validation 57, 62
vanity, all things are 11, 17–19, 21, 23, 26, 30, 35, 55, 57
virtue 1, 5, 6n6, 28, 38, 48, 69, 72

Watson, B. 20
Weeks, S. 6n2
well-being 47–48, 57, 67–68
wickedness 10, 21, 25
wisdom: abundance of 28, 36
wisdom *(Hokhmah):* abundance 36, 42; advantage of 12; failure of 35–36; futility of 5, 7, 32; inadequacies of 28, 35; and knowledge 19, 34; literature 3, 6n5; of love/love of 5; notion of 35; outlook on 39; poor man's 36; postmodern 14, 35, 80–81; writer 2, 12, 30
Wolf, Tom 1
women: dark view of 64–66, 72; love and marriage 66
work: calling 5, 57, 60; career 5, 60, 63n1; enjoyment from 74; meaning of 57; necessary evil 58–59; *see also* toil
workaholism 12, 56
worldview (Weltanschauung) 7–9, 15n2, 66, 77
Wrzesniewski A. (et al 1997) 63n3
wu-wei (inaction) 20

Zimmermann, F. 39n4

For Product Safety Concerns and Information please contact our EU representative GPSR@taylorandfrancis.com
Taylor & Francis Verlag GmbH, Kaufingerstraße 24, 80331 München, Germany

www.ingramcontent.com/pod-product-compliance
Ingram Content Group UK Ltd.
Pitfield, Milton Keynes, MK11 3LW, UK
UKHW022040111225
465993UK00009B/1006
* 9 7 8 1 0 4 1 0 9 9 7 6 5 *